The Pharmacy Technician Series

FUNDAMENTALS OF PHARMACY PRACTICE

Series Author
Mike Johnston, CPhT

Contributing Authors
Cliff Frank, CPhT
Robin Luke, CPhT

PEARSON
Prentice Hall

Upper Saddle River, New Jersey 07458

The Pharmacy Technician Series

The Pharmacy Technician Series

The Pharmacy Technician Series

The Pharmacy Technician Series

The Pharmacy Technician Series

Library of Congress Cataloging-in-Publication Data

The pharmacy technician series. Fundamentals of pharmacy practice / [edited by] Mike Johnston.
    p.   cm.
  Includes bibliographical references and index.
  ISBN 0-13-114751-X
  1. Pharmacy—Practice. 2. Pharmacy technicians. I. Title: Fundamentals of pharmacy practice.
  II. Johnston, Mike, CPhT.
  [DNLM: 1. Pharmacy—methods. 2. Pharmaceutical Preparations. 3. Technology, Pharmaceutical.
  QV 704 P5458 2006]
RS100.P494 2006
615'.1—dc22   2005045916

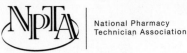

National Pharmacy
Technician Association

The NPTA logo is a trademark of the
National Pharmacy Technician Association

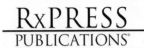

RxPRESS
PUBLICATIONS

The Straden-Schaden and RxPress logos are
both trademarks of Straden-Schaden, Inc.

Publisher: Julie Levin Alexander
Assistant to Publisher: Regina Bruno
Acquisitions Editor: Joan Gill
Developmental Editor: Triple SSS Press Media Development, Inc.
Editorial Assistant: Bronwen Glowacki
Director of Marketing: Karen Allman
Marketing Coordinator: Michael Sirinides
Channel Marketing Manager: Rachele Strober
Director of Production and Manufacturing: Bruce Johnson
Managing Production Editor: Patrick Walsh
Production Liaison: Christina Zingone
Production Editor: Rosaria Cassinese/Prepare, Inc.
Manufacturing Manager: Ilene Sanford
Manufacturing Buyer: Pat Brown
Design Director: Cheryl Asherman
Interior Designer: Amy Rosen
Cover Designer: Mary Siener
Cover Illustrator: Edward Sherman
Compositor: Prepare, Inc.
Printer/Binder: Courier/Kendallville
Cover Printer: Phoenix Color Corp.
Photo Acknowledgment: We wish to thank the National Pharmacy
  Technician Association, Multi Med Media, and Jeremy Van Pelt
  (photographer).

Cover Illustration: © 2006 by Edward Sherman

Notice: The author and the publisher of this volume have taken care to make certain that the doses of drugs and schedules of treatment are correct and compatible with the standards generally accepted at the time of publication. Nevertheless, as new information becomes available, changes in treatment and in the use of drugs become necessary. The reader is advised to carefully consult the instruction and information material included in the package insert of each drug or therapeutic agent before administration. This advise is especially important when using, administering, or recommending new and infrequently used drugs. The author and publisher disclaim all responsibility for any liability, loss, injury, or damage incurred as a consequence, directly or indirectly, of the use and application of any of the contents of this volume. It is the responsibility of the reader to familiarize himself or herself with the policies and procedures set by the federal, state, and local agencies as well as the institution or agency where the reader may be employed. It is the reader's responsibility to stay informed of any new changes or recommendations made by any federal, state, and local agency as well as by his or her employing institution or agency.

PEARSON
Prentice
Hall

10 9 8 7 6 5 4 3 2
ISBN 0-13-114751-X

Dedication

To my mother—*you are a strong woman; I am proud to have you as my mother. You provided our family comfort, security, and love and a childhood that not all are blessed enough to experience—but you ensured that I did.*

"I regard no man as poor who has a godly mother."—Abraham Lincoln.

To my father—*It is my hope that I can grow to become half the man you are. We never had to discuss how a respectable man lives and works, because I simply watched you. It makes me proud to share your name.*

"One father is more than a hundred schoolmasters."—George Herbert.

Contents

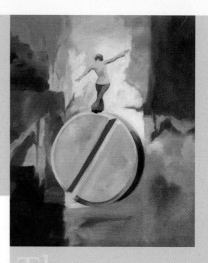

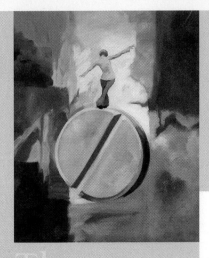

3 ## Terminology and Abbreviations 21

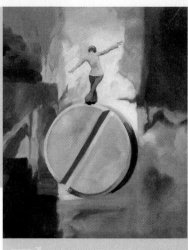

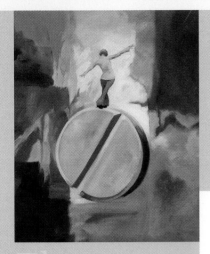

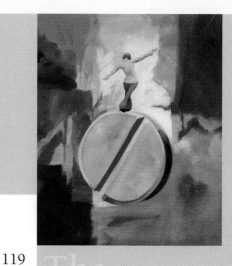

The
Pharmacy
Technician
Series

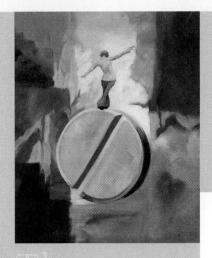

8   Community Pharmacy Calculations   141

9   Introduction to Compounding   151

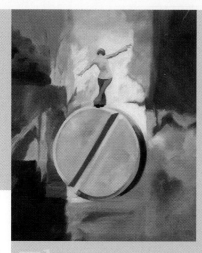

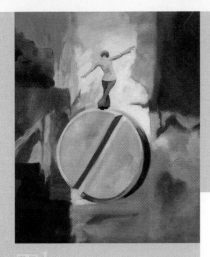

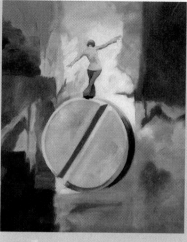

The Pharmacy Technician Series

The Pharmacy Technician Series

The Pharmacy Technician Series

The Pharmacy Technician Series

Preface

Fundamentals of Pharmacy Practice is the central title in Prentice Hall's newest series for pharmacy technician education. *The Pharmacy Technician Series* consists of six books that have been developed and designed together, ensuring greater success for the pharmacy technician student.

About the Book

The practice of pharmacy is exciting and rewarding; however, it is also complex, diverse, and demanding. This book has been designed to guide students through with ease, while building a solid foundation of knowledge for their careers.

The core features of this book include the following:

- Chapter introductions and summaries, which provide the student with a clearer understanding and rationale of the content being covered.
- *Workplace Wisdom* boxes offer quick highlighted tips and comments that replicate the advice of a seasoned pharmacy technician.

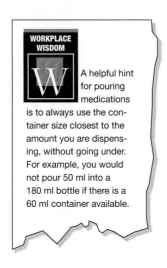

WORKPLACE WISDOM

A helpful hint for pouring medications is to always use the container size closest to the amount you are dispensing, without going under. For example, you would not pour 50 ml into a 180 ml bottle if there is a 60 ml container available.

• Profiles of Practice provide practical exercises that simulate "real world" pharmacy problems and give the student the opportunity to assess their knowledge.

PROFILES
OF PRACTICE

Can you decipher the sample prescriptions in Figures 7-6 through 7-8?

What is wrong with the prescriptions in Figure 7-9 and Figure 7-10?

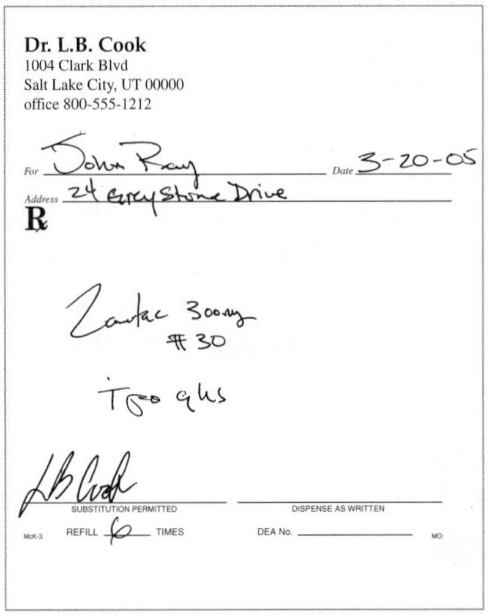

Dr. L.B. Cook
1004 Clark Blvd
Salt Lake City, UT 00000
office 800-555-1212

For _John Ray_   Date _3-20-05_
Address _24 Greystone Drive_
R

Zantac 300mg
#30

T po qhs

LB Cook
SUBSTITUTION PERMITTED   DISPENSE AS WRITTEN
McK-3   REFILL _6_ TIMES   DEA No. _____   MD

Figure 7-6   Sample prescription.

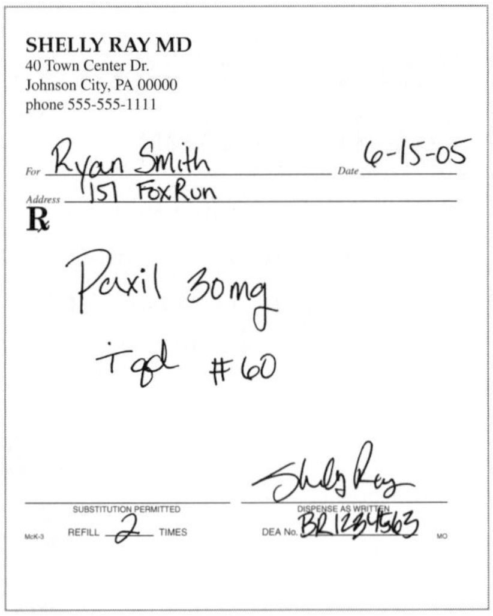

SHELLY RAY MD
40 Town Center Dr.
Johnson City, PA 00000
phone 555-555-1111

For _Ryan Smith_   Date _6-15-05_
Address _151 FoxRun_
R

Paxil 30mg
T qd #60

Shelly Ray
SUBSTITUTION PERMITTED   DISPENSE AS WRITTEN
McK-3   REFILL _2_ TIMES   DEA No. _BR 1234563_   MD

Figure 7-7   Sample prescription.

- Chapter Reviews present a learning assessment for both the student and the instructors to evaluate concept comprehension.

CHAPTER REVIEW QUESTIONS

1. Which of the following is not an example of ambulatory or retail pharmacy?
   a. franchise or chain pharmacy
   b. nursing home pharmacy
   c. privately owned pharmacy
   d. All of the above are examples.

2. The term "ambulatory pharmacy" refers to a setting in which:
   a. the patient arrives by ambulance.
   b. the patient lives at the facility where the pharmacy is located.
   c. the patient walks into the pharmacy.
   d. the pharmacy is part of a larger facility.

3. Which of the following does not need to be recorded on a prescription?

6. Which of the following tasks may a technician not perform?
   a. fill a prescription from a fax
   b. accept a refill order from a patient
   c. accept a prescription order by phone
   d. call an insurer on behalf of a patient

7. Before selecting the medication to fill an order, a technician should:
   a. check the brand name
   b. check the NDC and/or UPC code
   c. check the contraindications
   d. check with the pharmacist

8. Which of the following does not appear on the patient's bottle?
   a. name of the medication being dispensed

- Top 200 Drugs is a current listing of the most prescribed medications in the United States. The drugs are categorized by their generic names trade names, classes and uses, available strengths, and dosage forms.
- Professional Resources Appendix—students will depend on this text for years, as it contains the most comprehensive published list of professional resources specifically for pharmacy technicians, including books, certification, accreditation, regulations, professional organizations, and government agencies.

About the Series

While there has been a variety of textbooks and training manuals for pharmacy technician education available, none has met the true educational needs of the industry—until now.

We set out to develop the most comprehensive, accurate, and current texts ever published for pharmacy technicians. One method we used to achieve this goal was involving pharmacy technician educators and trainers from across the country in every phase of the project. You will find that each title in this series has been developed, written, and reviewed exclusively by practicing pharmacy technician educators and practicing pharmacy professionals—a winning approach.

About the Authors

Cliff Frank, CPhT

Cliff retired in 1990 from a long career in retail management and training. He then moved to Alaska with his wife and began a second career as a pharmacy technician, practicing in retail, home health care, and hospital settings. In 1998, Cliff developed a pharmacy technician training program for the University of Alaska in Anchorage and managed that program until 2004.

In 2003, Cliff was honored by NPTA as the Pharmacy Technician Advocate of the Year. Today Cliff serves as the Alaska State Coordinator of NPTA and is developing a new pharmacy technician training program to be implemented across his entire home state.

Robin Luke, CPhT

Robin is a founding member of NPTA's Executive Advisory Board, the elected body of leaders for the National Pharmacy Technician Association. She has over ten years of experience in institutional pharmacy, sterile product preparation, compounding, bulk-manufacturing, and management, with a specialized knowledge of herbals and homeopathic treatments.

Robin has developed a variety of continuing education programs with a strong emphasis on reducing medication errors; she also speaks at meetings and conferences across the United States.

with

Mike Johnston, CPhT

Mike is known internationally as a respected author and speaker in the field of pharmacy. He published his first book, *Rx for Success—A Career Enhancement Guide for Pharmacy Technicians*, in 2002.

In 1999, Mike founded NPTA in Houston, Texas, and led the association from 3 members to over 20,000 in less than two years. Today, as Executive Director of the National Pharmacy Technician Association and publisher of *Today's Technician* magazine, he spends the majority of his time meeting with and speaking to employers, manufacturers, association leaders, and elected officials on issues related to pharmacy technicians.

About NPTA

NPTA, the National Pharmacy Technician Association, is the world's largest professional organization established specifically for pharmacy technicians. The association is dedicated to advancing the value of pharmacy technicians and the vital roles they play in pharmaceutical care. In a society of countless associations, we believe it takes much more than a mission statement to meet the professional needs and provide the needed leadership for the pharmacy technician profession—it takes action and results.

The organization is composed of pharmacy technicians practicing in a variety of practice settings, such as: retail, independent, hospital, mail-order, home care, long-term care, nuclear, military, correctional facility, formal education, training, management, sales, and many more. NPTA is a reflection of this diverse profession and provides unparallel support and resources to members.

NPTA is The Foundation of the Pharmacy Technician Profession; we have an unprecedented past, a strong presence and a promising future. We are dedicated to improving our profession, while remaining focused on our members.

For more information on NPTA:
Call 888-247-8700
Visit www.pharmacytechnician.org

Acknowledgments

This book, which is part of a six-title series, has been both an exhilarating and an exhausting project. To say that this series is the result of a collaborative, team effort would be a gross understatement.

Special thanks to SaveWay Compounding Pharmacy (Bear, Delaware), PCCA (Professional Compounding Centers of America, Houston, Texas), and Clarian Health System (Indianapolis, Indiana) for your assistance with this text. Nearly every photograph presented throughout this book was shot on location at your facilities. We are grateful for the assistance, patience, and collaboration of your entire staff.

We would also like to thank Jeremy Van Pelt (Photographer) and Multi Med Media (Production Management).

Mark — thank you for believing in my initial vision and concept for this series, which was anything but traditional. I will always remember the day we spent in New York City talking about cover concepts and the like at coffee shops and art galleries. More importantly, I am honored to have gotten to know you, Alex, and now little Sophie—and I consider each of you as friends.

Joan — you are truly gifted at what you do. I am amazed at your ability to join this project at the point you did and to guide each daunting task to a smooth and successful accomplishment. I feel that your leadership has created a better final product.

Julie — thank you for taking risks (plural) on this project, boldly departing from standard policies and procedures. In the end, your support and belief in this project allowed a truly innovative product to be published.

Robin — your commitment to this project —to exceeding all expectations, to developing the best training series for pharmacy technicians available—has been amazing. You are a wonderful, gifted individual; but most importantly, I am thankful to call you a friend.

Andrew and Jenny — thank you for supporting this project, each in your own unique way; thank you for supporting me and the entire organization. This project tested each of us—our character and our will—and I am honored to know you both.

Most importantly, I wish to thank my family. The past several years have been difficult and trying, but the strength, love, and support that you have given me have always pulled me through. *Thank you.*

Contributors

Andrew Cordiale, CPhT
Assistant Title Manager
Glen Falls Hospital
Queensbury, NY

Mark Abell, PA
Lowell, FL

Jennifer Bissen, CPhT
Inteq, Inc.
Dallas, TX

Jennifer Fix, RPh, MBA
Haltom City, TX

Antoinette Iannuzzelli, CPhT
CVS/Pharmacy
Nutley, NJ

Brenda Pavlic, CPhT
Saveway Compounding Pharmacy
Bear, DE

Carol Reyes, CPhT
Oncology Specialists, S.C.
Franklin Park, IL

LaShara C. Smith, CPhT
Fletcher-Med Pharmacy
San Diego, CA

Evelyn White, CPhT
Apple Drug
Berlin, MD

Reviewers

The reviewers of *The Pharmacy Technician Series* have provided many excellent suggestions and ideas for improving these texts. The quality of the reviews has been outstanding, and the reviews have been a major aid in the preparation of the manuscript. The assistance provided by these experts is deeply appreciated.

Lisa C. Barnes, B. Pharm, M.B.A.
ACPE Program Administrator, Adjunct Assistant Professor of Pharmacy Practice
University of Montana School of Pharmacy and Allied Health Sciences
Missoula, Montana

Kimberly Brown, CPh.T.
Associate Director and Instructor of Pharmacy Technology
Walters State Community College
Morristown, Tennessee 37813

Ralph P. Casas, Pharm. D., Ph.D.
Associate Professor of Pharmacology
Cerritos Community College
Norwalk, California

Kristie Fitzgerald
Clinical Pharmacist, Department of Neonatology; Instructor
Salt Lake Community College
Salt Lake City, Utah

Madeline Jensen-Grauel, B.S., Ed., M.Sc.
Director, Pharmacy Technician Training Program
The University of Texas Medical Branch at Galveston
Galveston, Texas

Robert D. Kwiatkowski, B.S., M.A.
Adjunct Instructor
PIMA Medical Institute
Colorado Springs, Colorado

Herminio Maldonado, Jr., M.S., B.S.
Pharmacy Technician Instructor
PIMA Medical Institute
Colorado Springs, Colorado

Bradley Moore, MSN
Director of Health Science
Remington Administrative Services, Inc.
Little Rock, Arkansas

Hieu Nguyen, B.S., CPh.T.
Pharmacy Technician Program Director
Western Career College
Sacramento, California

History of Pharmacy Practice

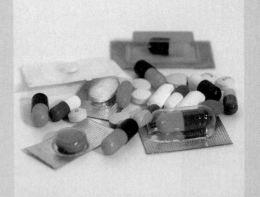

Learning Objectives

After completing this chapter, you
should be able to:

- Explain the origins of modern
  pharmacy practice.
- Compare and contrast modern
  and historic pharmacy practice.
- List some landmark references
  for pharmacy practitioners.

INTRODUCTION

Pharmacy is the science of preparing and dispensing
medications, as well as supplying drug-related information to
patients and consumers. Basically, the pharmacy team is
charged with the challenge of getting the right patient the
right medication in the right form and dose at the right time.
The practice of pharmacy, therefore, is directly related to the
fields of medicine and chemistry. It is incorporated into a
branch of the medical sciences called materia medica. This
area of science is concerned with the sources, nature,
properties, and preparations of drugs.

Pharmacy is also deeply immersed in the larger field of health
care. In modern times, changes in health care have accelerated
rapidly and show no signs of slowing down. The pharmacy
technician is a relatively recent addition to the health care team
and is a position growing in scope, as well as in practice. In short,
the role and responsibilities of pharmacy technicians continue to
change dramatically, and thus there is a serious need for
education and training. With the support of well-trained and
educated technicians, the pharmacist is able to devote the
required time and effort to patient counseling, drug utilization
review, and consultations with other health care providers.

Evolution of Pharmacy Practice

In order to understand the pharmacy practices of the modern world, it is necessary to first explore the history of pharmacy. By doing this, we will have a greater understanding of the beginnings and evolution of the practice of pharmacy.

Originally, the field of pharmacy was combined with both medicine and religion. Men and women who practiced pharmacy often administered religious rites as well. These were the medicine men, shamans, and religious leaders of their communities. This association remained imbedded in pharmacy for hundreds of years.

Specialization of pharmacy as a profession first began in the eighth century in an area that is now known as Baghdad. The occupation of pharmacy progressively spread to Europe and took on the name *alchemy*. Alchemy eventually evolved, with the help of the physicians of the time, into what we know as chemistry. In fact, in Australia today, the pharmacist is still known as a chemist.

The physicians of antiquity often not only diagnosed their patients, but also prescribed and dispensed the medications. Over time, there grew a need for specialists who would be able to compound the medications in bulk. About the year 1200, Frederick the Great decreed the first pharmacy law separating the profession of medicine from the profession of pharmacy. Hence, the field we know as pharmacy grew even further and began to include the compounding of medications and remedies for the general public. The medications that became available were known as elixirs, spirits, and powders. No one regulated the formulas, manufacture, or dispensing of any of these medications until centuries later.

As time passed, the line between physicians and pharmacists became more defined. Publications arose called Pharmacopeias. The first ones were the *Pharmacopeia of London* (1618) and the *Pharmacopeia of Paris* (1639). In these journals were lists of medications, elixirs, and other remedies of the time. They were recipe books, if you will.

In the United States, circa 1820, the first publication concerning pharmacy was written. This was called the *Pharmacopeia of the United States*. This is still an ongoing publication used by pharmacists and other health care professionals today. Selections for this resource are made by a group of individuals who make up the Committee on Revision. These committee members include the Surgeon General of the United States, representatives of all colleges of medicine and pharmacy, as well as representatives of all state medical and pharmaceutical associations.

CONCLUSION

As has been explained in this historical overview of pharmacy practices, the pharmaceutical field has become highly regulated and much larger in scope over time. Legislation and regulatory organizations are a dominant factor, but so is the growing need for safe, effective, and affordable health care. The field of pharmacy is very challenging and rewarding: but before an individual decides to enter this field, a proper education and knowledge base are required.

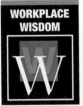
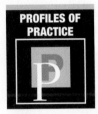

CHAPTER REVIEW QUESTIONS

1. Why should you keep current in your skills and knowledge of pharmacy?
   a. The pharmacy profession is ever evolving.
   b. New medications come out practically weekly.
   c. Keep current with continuing education needs.
   d. all of the above

2. Pharmacy was originally mixed in with what?
   a. religion
   b. politics
   c. agriculture
   d. mathematics

3. Pharmacy is incorporated in a branch of the medical sciences called:
   a. medicinal management
   b. materia medica
   c. montria moderna
   d. motronial medici

4. The *Pharmacopeia* originally came from London in:
   a. 1816
   b. 1734
   c. 1200
   d. 1618

5. The *Pharmacopeia of the United States* is:
   a. an historical relic
   b. still used today
   c. no longer used
   d. used in some schools

Resources and References

1. Reifman, Noah. *Certification Review for Pharmacy Technicians, 6th Ed.* Evergreen, CO: Ark Pharmaceutical Consultants, Inc., 2002.
2. American Pharmacist Association. *Pharmacy Technician Workbook and Certification Review.* Englewood, CO: Morton Publishing, 2001.
3. American Society of Health System Pharmacists. *Manual for Pharmacy Technicians.* Bethesda, MD: ASHP, 1998.
4. American Society of Health System Pharmacists. *Pharmacy Technician Certification Review and Exam.* Bethesda, MD: ASHP, 1998.
5. Ballington, Don. *Pharmacy Practice.* St. Paul, MN: EMC Paradigm, 1999.
6. Ballington, Don. *Pharmacy Practice for Technicians.* St. Paul, MN: EMC Paradigm, 2003.
7. Cowen, D. and W. Helfand. *Pharmacy: An Illustrated History.* New York: Harry N. Abrams, Incorporated, 1990.
8. Lambert, Anita. *Advanced Pharmacy Practice for Technicians.* Clifton Park, NY: Delmar, 2002.
9. American Pharmacist Association. *The Pharmacy Technician.* 2nd Ed. Englewood, CO: Morton Publishing, 2004.

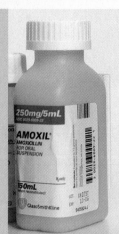

CHAPTER 2

Pharmacy Law and Ethics

INTRODUCTION

Federal and state laws, as well as professional ethics, regulate the practice of pharmacy. The regulations on pharmacy practice in the United States have evolved and increased over the past 100 years, as legislators respond to outcries from citizens to serve and protect the public interest. The government began to take the initiative in the regulatory affairs of pharmacy at the end of the 18th century. As time has passed, the profession of pharmacy has acquired more regulations than were ever thought possible back in the 1800s. In the United States, a professional degree is a requirement for any individual who wishes to practice pharmacy. This requirement was established to protect the public and set minimal standards that the citizens could rely upon.

In this chapter you will focus primarily on the major federal regulations pertaining to pharmacy practice; but please note that this chapter does not list all federal laws pertaining to pharmacy, all regulations included in the laws presented, or state regulations.

Ethics and the Pharmacy Technician

As in many professions, ethics is a factor in decision making for pharmacy professionals, including pharmacy technicians. Many situations can and will arise in which you or your colleagues will be required to make ethical decisions. Ethical decisions are those grey areas where there is no clear-cut, black or white, correct or incorrect response or decision. These decisions require an understanding of a professional code of ethics, as well as an understanding of moral principles and their application to your own life. Ethics is not law, religion, or morals, but all of these can affect your ethical decisions. Ethics is as personal as your individual faith and covers much of your behavior. In a profession, there is often an ethical code adopted by members of that profession. This code can serve as a guidepost or parameter to aid you in your reasoning process when a decision is required. Keeping your ethical decisions within the limits of an ethical code can also serve you if you are called upon to defend your actions. Consider the following scenario: Mrs. Mortimer, a regular customer, arrives at your pharmacy and demands a refill for her synthroid. While processing her order, you discover that she has no refills left on her prescription. It is 9 p.m. on Friday night, and Monday is the Fourth of July. You notify the pharmacist of the situation and await further instructions. As another scenario, consider the distribution problem that arises when there is a vaccine or medication shortage.

Several moral principles concern pharmacy professionals. These principles are the basis for the theories of ethical practice discussed next. While reviewing the principles, keep in mind that there may be conflicts between them. For instance, beneficence may help the most people, but requires abandoning veracity. Here are the five principles:

- beneficence—bringing about good
- fidelity—promise keeping
- veracity—telling the truth
- justice—acting with fairness or equity within the law
- autonomy—acting with self-reliance

Defining Ethics

Ethics is commonly defined as the considered reflection and systematic analysis of the morality of certain behavior when required actions are unclear. An ethical decision is not an emotional, knee-jerk reaction, therefore, but something that has been weighed and measured carefully.

Moral Philosophy

The moral reasoning process that attempts to help you decide the rightness or wrongness of conduct (a value system, if you will) is your moral philosophy. This philosophy will guide you in reaching ethical decisions that further your professional goals.

Practicing Ethics

The next step is measuring a certain conduct against a value system. Defending that conduct is critical to ethical practice, which, as you remember, is "to be good and to act well."

Ethical Theories

The following nine theories can help you measure possible ethical decisions.

CONSEQUENTIALISM

"The purpose of all actions should be to bring about the greatest good to the greatest number." Do you think Mrs. Mortimer's situation could be applied here? What about restricting the use of flu vaccine in the case of a medication shortage? How could that decision be guided under this theory?

NONCONSEQUENTIALISM

"Nonconsequentialism is the study of actions themselves without regard to outcome." Could the pharmacist argue that Mrs. Mortimer having her medication is more important than the law that says legend drugs cannot be dispensed without a valid prescription? In the case of a shortage, could we say that first come–first served is the fairest way to distribute vaccine?

SOCIAL CONTRACTS

"Pharmacists, technicians, and patients recognize certain expectations of each other and act accordingly." Can Mrs. Mortimer argue that she entrusts the pharmacist with the responsibility to provide for her medication needs? Could the pharmacist in turn argue that her dilemma is not his problem, because Mrs. Mortimer has a responsibility to keep her prescriptions current and he in turn should expect such behavior? How would this theory apply to the vaccine situation?

THE ETHICS OF CARE

"This principle requires the decision-maker to more clearly focus on such basic moral skills as kindness, sensitivity, attentiveness, tact, patience, and reliability." Should the pharmacist ask himself what the kind and reliable action would be? Could he argue that "teaching" Mrs. Mortimer to be more conscientious by refusing to fill her expired prescription would be the better path? What is the most humane action in the face of a vaccine shortage?

RIGHTS-BASED ETHICS

This theory is based on an understanding of human rights—the belief that an individual in a democratic society should be shielded from undue forces and allowed to enjoy and pursue personal projects; that is, the individual has certain "rights," legal as well as moral. Does Mrs. Mortimer have a right to her medication despite any rules or regulations? Could the pharmacist argue that he should fill her prescription because it is her right? How would rights-based ethics apply to the vaccine shortage?

PRINCIPLE-BASED ETHICS

"Moral principles are general, universal guides to action." This is a more personal approach. The pharmacist could say that going against a law for him is immoral. It could also be argued that refusing medication to anyone who needs it is also immoral. You could ask, Is it ever moral to deny medication to anyone in need? How does that change in a shortage situation?

VIRTUE-BASED ETHICS

"The use of virtues in establishing right reason in action." In Mrs. Mortimer's case, what would the most virtuous action be? What about in the vaccine shortage case?

LAW

Law is closely related to the system of ethics and sometimes overlaps it, creating confusion and tension about the "right thing to do" in a given situation. Mrs. Mortimer is a good example. The laws governing prescriptions are very clear. They do not allow for exceptions. The pharmacist could definitely quote the law to Mrs. Mortimer and refuse to fill her prescription, arguing that the law is the law and his hands are tied. Are there any laws governing the distribution of drugs? Would they apply to the vaccine case? Should there be new laws for just such a case?

CODES OF ETHICS

"An identifying benchmark for all professions is their sincere acceptance of the responsibility to maintain a standard of conduct beyond either an unthinking conformity to the law or the routine performance of technical skill." The code of ethics that follows is an example of the ninth ethical theory. It was written by technicians for technicians and adopted by the American Association of Pharmacy Technicians in 1996. Can you find an answer to Mrs. Mortimer's dilemma here that would work for you?

Pharmacy Technician Code of Ethics (1996)

Pharmacy technicians are health care professionals who assist pharmacists in providing the best possible care for patients. The principles of this code, which apply to pharmacy technicians working in any and all settings, are based on the application and support of the moral obligations that guide the pharmacy profession in relationships with patients, health care professionals, and society.

PREAMBLE

I. A pharmacy technician's first considerations are to ensure the health and safety of the patient and to use knowledge and skills to the best of his ability in serving others.

II. A pharmacy technician supports and promotes honesty and integrity in the profession, which includes a duty to observe the law, maintain the highest moral and ethical conduct at all times, and uphold the ethical principles of the profession.

III. A pharmacy technician assists and supports the pharmacist in the safe, efficacious, and cost-effective distribution of health services and health care resources.

IV. A pharmacy technician respects and values the abilities of pharmacists, colleagues, and other health care professionals.

V. A pharmacy technician maintains competency in his practice, and continually enhances his professional knowledge and expertise.

VI. A pharmacy technician respects and supports the patient's individuality, dignity, and confidentiality.

VII. A pharmacy technician respects the confidentiality of the patient's records and discloses pertinent information only with proper authorization.

VIII. A pharmacy technician never assists in the dispensing or distributing of medications or medical devices that are not of good quality or do not meet the standards required by law.

IX. A pharmacy technician does not engage in any activity that will discredit the profession, and he will expose, without fear or favor, illegal or unethical conduct in the profession.

X. A pharmacy technician associates with and engages in the support of organizations that promote the profession of pharmacy through the use and enhancement of pharmacy technicians.

Overview of Pharmacy Law

The public's concern over the sulfanilamide disaster (see "Profiles of Practice" near the end of the chapter) is an example of the kinds of events that have prompted lawmakers to draft new legislation governing the safety of drugs.

FDCA—FOOD, DRUG, AND COSMETIC ACT

In 1938, U.S. legislators passed the Food, Drug, and Cosmetic Act, commonly referred to as the FDCA. The purpose of the FDCA was to limit interstate commerce in drugs to those that are safe and effective. Among the many major provisions of this legislation were the following:

- Manufacturers were required to submit evidence that new drugs were safe prior to marketing.

- All drugs had to have warnings and adequate directions for use.
- New drugs were required to be tested clinically before being marketed to the public.
- Drugs used as diagnostic agents, therapeutic devices, and cosmetics were regulated for the first time.

The FDCA established an agency within the U.S. Department of Health and Human Services to oversee the new policies: the FDA, or Food and Drug Administration.

Many of the provisions of the FDCA pertain to requirements for the label of the drug. It is important to understand and recognize the difference between the label of a drug and the labeling of a drug. While these sound the same, they are actually two uniquely different components regulated under the FDCA. The label of a drug refers to "a display of written, printed, or graphic matter upon the immediate container of any article; it is the information on the outer portion of the package or container. The labeling of a drug refers to "all labels and other written, printed, or graphic[al matter] either upon or accompanying the drug." The labeling is broader in scope than the label; the labeling of a drug includes the label, as well as package inserts.

The FDCA also regulated who could prescribe legend drugs. The FDCA does not require that the prescriber be licensed in the state where the prescription is actually filled, so long as the prescription is valid in the state it was written in. A prescriber is permitted to delegate an authorized individual to transmit a prescription; however, the prescriber cannot delegate the authority to prescribe or authorize a refill.

There have been numerous amendments to the original FDCA of 1938, as well as related legislative acts. While this text will not cover all of these amendments and acts, several of the most prominent ones will be described.

Durham-Humphrey Amendment of 1951

Also known as the Prescription Drug Amendment, the Durham-Humphrey Amendment of 1951 required that prescription drugs bear the legend, "Caution: Federal law prohibits dispensing without a prescription." This required legend is the reason why prescription drugs are referred to as legend drugs. Later amendments approved a substitute legend that simply reads "RX only."

Kefauver-Harris Amendments of 1962

Also known as the Drug Efficacy Amendments, the Kefauver-Harris Amendments of 1962 focused on accountability from drug manufacturers for the efficacy, or effectiveness, of drugs. Several provisions of these amendments include the following:

- Good Manufacturing Practices (GMP) were established for manufacturers.
- Prior to marketing any new drug, manufacturers were required to supply proof of effectiveness and safety.
- Advertising of prescription drugs was placed under the supervision of the FDA.

- Procedures for new drug applications and investigational drugs were established.

Drug Abuse Control Amendments of 1965

The Drug Abuse Control Amendments of 1965 provided the first guidelines for determining the classification of drugs subject to abuse.

Comprehensive Drug Abuse Prevention and Control Act of 1970

In 1970, the Comprehensive Drug Abuse Prevention and Control Act essentially combined all of the federal laws dealing with narcotics, stimulants, depressants, and abused designer drugs.

Medical Device Amendment of 1976

This amendment required for the first time that the safety and effectiveness of life-sustaining and life-supporting devices have premarket approval of the FDA.

Legend Drugs—Prescribing and Dispensing

According to the FDCA, legend drugs may be prescribed only by a practitioner licensed to administer and prescribe such drugs. Such practitioners may include physicians, surgeons, veterinarians, dentists, physician assistants, nurse practitioners, and even pharmacists in certain states and according to specific regulations.

The preceding laws and regulations govern drugs dispensed for human use, but be aware that additional or modified requirements are in place for drugs dispensed for animal use.

Labeling requirements for dispensed prescriptions include the following (Figure 2-1):

- pharmacy name and address
- serial number (Rx Number)
- date of fill
- expiration date
- prescriber's name
- patient's name
- directions for use
- cautionary statements (if needed)

OTC Drugs

The FDCA requires that drugs approved for over-the-counter (OTC) distribution include the following information on the label of the drug (Figure 2-2):

- the product's name
- the name and address of the manufacturer, distributor, repacker, and so on

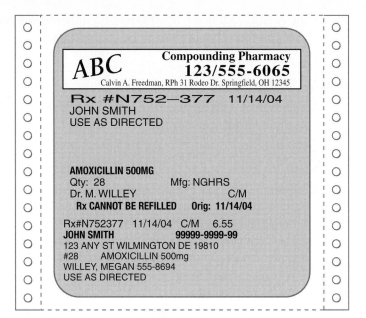

Figure 2-1 A sample prescription label

Drug Facts

Active Ingredient (in each geltab)   **Purpose**
Acetaminophen 500 mg .... Analgesic & Antipyretic

Uses for temporary relief of minor aches and pains associated with:
- headache
- minor arthritis pain
- muscular aches
- backache
- common cold
- menstrual cramps
- toothache
- reduction of fever

Warnings
Alcohol Warning: If you generally consume 3 or more alcoholic drinks every day, ask your doctor whether you should take acetaminophen or other pain relievers/fever reducers. Acetaminophen may cause liver damage.
Overdose Warning: Taking more than the recommended dose (overdose) could cause serious health problems. In case of overdose, get medical help or contact a Poison Control Center right away. Prompt medical attention is critical in adults as well as children even if you do not notice any signs or symptoms.
Do not exceed recommended dosage.   ▼

Drug Facts (continued)
Do not use ■ with other products containing acetaminophen ■ for more than 10 days for pain unless directed by a doctor ■ for more than 3 days for fever unless directed by a doctor
Stop use and ask a doctor if
- symptoms do not improve
- any new or unexpected symptoms occur
- redness or swelling is present
- pain or fever persists or gets worse

If pregnant or breast-feeding, ask a health professional before use. **Keep out of reach of children.**

Directions **Adults and children 12 years of age and over:** take 2 geltabs every 4 to 6 hours. Do not exceed 8 geltabs in 24 hours, or as directed by your doctor. **Children under 12 years of age:** do not use this product in children under 12 years of age. This will provide more than the recommended dose (overdose) and could cause serious health problems.

Other information ■ store at controlled room temperature 15°-30°C (59°-86°F) ■ do not use if imprinted safety seal under cap is broken or missing.   ▼

Drug Facts (continued)
Inactive ingredients Carnauba wax, D&C Yellow #10 Lake, FD&C Red #40 Aluminum Lake, gelatin, glycerin, hypromellose, polyethylene glycol, povidone, starch, purified water, sodium starch glycolate, stearic acid, titanium dioxide. May also contain: microcrystalline cellulose.

*This product is not manufactured or distributed by McNeil Consumer Healthcare, owner of the registered trademark TYLENOL®.
Distributed by: Walgreen Co., Deerfield, IL 60015-4616
100% Satisfaction Guaranteed www.walgreens.com

Figure 2-2 A sample OTC label (*Courtesy of Walgreen Co.*)

- the established name of all active ingredients and the quantities of certain other ingredients (active or inactive)
- the net contents
- required cautions and warnings
- the name of any habit-forming drug contained in the formula
- adequate directions for use

PPPA

According to the Poison Prevention Packaging Act, all legend and controlled drugs, with some exceptions, must be dispensed in a childproof container. For patients such as the elderly, who do not wish to have their medications dispensed in such containers, a signed, written request should be kept on file at the pharmacy. Exceptions to the PPPA include sublingual doses of nitroglycerin, contraceptives, drugs dispensed to inpatients in hospitals, and certain emergency medications.

The FDCA requires that legend, or prescription-only, drugs include the following information on the label of the drug (Figure 2-3):

- its established name and quantity of each active ingredient
- statement of new quantity
- statement of usual dosage
- federal legend
- route of administration
- in the case of habit-forming drugs, the federal warning
- name of all inactive ingredients, if intended for route of administration other than oral
- a unique lot or control number
- a statement specifying the type of container to be used in dispensing
- the name and place of business of the manufacturer, packer, or distributor
- an expiration date, if applicable

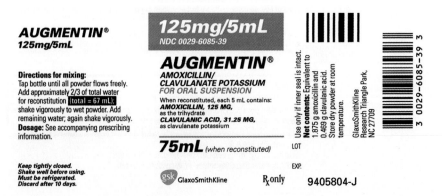

Figure 2-3 An example of a legend drug product label (*Courtesy of GlaxoSmithKline*)

While the label is considered a component of the labeling of a drug, the FDA also requires additional information to accompany the legend drug on its labeling. The following information is required by the FDA and is usually provided in the package insert:

- description, which is usually a chemical structure
- clinical pharmacology
- indications and usage
- contraindications—situations in which the drug should not be used
- warnings—side effects and potential safety hazards
- precautions—detailed special care that must be taken by the prescriber
- adverse reactions
- drug abuse and dependence
- dosage
- statement as to how supplied
- the date of the most recent revision to the labeling

ADULTERATION VERSUS MISBRANDING

According to the FDA, an adulterated drug is a drug that is in a condition contrary to the intentions of the manufacturer; adulteration focuses on the physical condition of the drug or device. On the other hand, misbranding focuses on the representations made by the manufacturer. Following are some criteria, any one of which is sufficient for constituting adulteration or misbranding:

Adulterated Drugs

- are prepared, packed, or held under unsanitary conditions
- are manufactured in a way that does not conform with the established GMP
- have a container composed of a poisonous or deleterious substance
- contain an unsafe color additive
- vary from an official compendium standard
- are new, unsafe, animal drugs or animal feeds containing such drugs
- are a class III device without premarket approval—a banned device
- are OTC drugs that are not packaged in tamper-resistant packaging

Misbranded Drugs

- have false or misleading labels
- have labels that fail to state the name and place of business of the manufacturer, packer, or distributor and that lack an accurate statement of quantity
- have labels with required information that is not prominently placed on them

- have labels that do not state "Warning: May Be Habit Forming" in the case of habit-forming substances
- have labels that, in the case of legend drugs, do not include the generic name or the names of ingredients, or the type on the label is not less than one-half the size of the trade/brand name
- are listed in an official compendium (unless they are labeled and packed by compendium standards)
- are in packages that are misleading
- are subject to deterioration, and the label does not bear corresponding precautionary statements
- endanger one's health if used in the manner suggested by the labeling
- are composed of either insulin or an antibiotic drug and are not batch certified
- contain a color additive and are not labeled accordingly
- are produced by manufacturers who are not registered with the FDA and who do not list the drug as one they manufacture
- are subject to the Poison Prevention Packaging Act of 1970 and are not packaged accordingly
- are touted in advertisements that fail to mention the generic or established names (if they are prescription drugs) and that omit the side effects, warnings, contraindications, effectiveness, and quantitative formulas of the drugs
- have labels with inadequate directions for their use and inadequate warnings about their effects
- have labels that fail to bear the statement "Caution: Federal law restricts this drug to use by or on the order of a licensed veterinarian" in the case of veterinary drugs

NEW DRUGS

According to the FDCA, there are in essence only two ways in which drugs can be lawfully sold in the United States. The drug must either be exempted through the 1962 amendments or be approved by the FDA under the procedures for a new drug application.

The process by which the FDA approves new drugs includes the approval of an investigational new drug (IND) through the filing of a new drug application (NDA). This process can take years before gaining approval, if ever, not counting the many years of research and development.

SAMPLES

The following are considered drug samples by the FDA: any drug that is habit forming, bears the federal legend or is restricted to investigational use and that is not intended to be sold, but rather to promote the sale of the drug.

Manufacturers and distributors are permitted by the FDA to distribute drug samples upon written request of a prescriber and under a system that requires the recipient to execute a written receipt for the sample and return the receipt to the manufacturer.

MEDICAL DEVICES

A medical device is an instrument or machine that is recognized in either the National Formulary or *U.S. Pharmacopoeia*. It is intended for the diagnosis, cure, mitigation, treatment or prevention of disease, or it is intended to affect the structure or any function of the body of a human or animal.

The FDCA categorizes medical devices by three classes. Class I devices are those that have relatively low potential for causing harm, such as scissors or needles. Class II devices require specific performance standards established by a panel of experts. Examples of Class II devices include thermometers, hearing aids, and catheters. Class III medical devices are life-supporting systems whose failure could cause death or serious injury.

CSA—CONTROLLED SUBSTANCES ACT

The Controlled Substances Act of 1970 established five classes, referred to as schedules, for controlled substances. These schedules represent the potential for abuse for each drug. This legislation was enacted to ensure the safety of the public. The schedules range from I to V.

Schedule I

These drugs have a high potential for abuse. They have no currently accepted medical use in the United States, or there is a lack of an accepted safety standard for use of the drug. Examples of drugs in Schedule I include heroin, LSD, and marijuana. C-I is the symbol for this class of drugs.

Schedule II

These drugs have a currently accepted medical use in the United States, but they have a high potential for abuse, or the abuse of the drug or other substance may lead to severe dependence. Examples of drugs in Schedule II include cocaine, morphine, and Ritalin®. C-II is the symbol for this class of drugs.

Schedule III

These drugs have less potential for abuse than those in Schedules I and II, have a currently accepted medical use in the United States, or the abuse of these drugs may lead to moderate physical dependence or high psychological dependence. Examples of drugs in Schedule III include Noludar® and anabolic steroids. C-III is the symbol for this class of drugs. Schedule III substances may be refilled if authorized by the prescriber; however, refills are limited to five times and must be filled within six months of the date issued.

Schedule IV

These drugs have a low potential for abuse, have a currently accepted medical use in the United States, or the abuse of these drugs may lead to limited dependence. Examples include Vicodin®, Valium®, and Librium®. C-IV is the symbol for this class of drugs. Schedule IV substances may be refilled if authorized by the prescriber; however, refills are limited to five times and must be filled within six months of the date issued.

Schedule V

These drugs have a low potential for abuse, have a currently accepted medical use in the United States, or the abuse of these drugs may lead to limited dependence in relation to all other controlled substances. An example of a Schedule V drug is Lomotil®. C-V is the symbol for this class of drugs. Schedule V substances do not have additional requirements on refills, and can be refilled for one year according to the prescriber's directions.

The DEA

The Controlled Substances Act established the Drug Enforcement Administration (DEA), which is an agency within the U.S. Department of Justice. It is a closed system, as the distribution of controlled substances is only permitted between those entities registered with the DEA.

The DEA regulates the legal trade in narcotic and dangerous drugs, manages a national narcotics intelligence system, and works with other agencies to support drug traffic prevention. In 1982, synchronized jurisdiction over drug offenses was given to the Federal Bureau of Investigation (FBI) and the DEA. Agents of the two organizations work together on drug law enforcement, and the DEA's administrator reports to the director of the FBI. The DEA has offices nationwide and in more than 40 foreign countries.

Activities Requiring DEA Approval

Participating in any of the following activities requires registration with the DEA:

- manufacturing controlled substances
- distributing controlled substances
- dispensing controlled substances
- conducting research with controlled substances
- conducting instructional activities with controlled substances
- conducting a narcotic treatment program
- conducting chemical analysis with controlled substances
- importing or exporting controlled substances
- compounding controlled substances

Those who engage in any of these activities must register with the DEA, using either Form 225 (to manufacture or distribute), Form 224 (to dispense), or Form 363 (to compound or conduct a narcotic treatment program). Initial registration is granted for a period of 28 to 39 months, after which the registration period is every 36 months.

Registrants (those who are approved by the DEA) receive a unique identification number, referred to as their DEA number, to be used within the closed system.

Prescribing and Dispensing Controlled Substances

According to the CSA, prescriptions for controlled substances are required to include the folowing:

- the full name and address of the patient
- the name, address, and registry number of the prescriber
- the date issued
- a manual signature of the prescriber

In addition, prescriptions for controlled substances are required to be written in ink or by a typewriter or an indelible pencil.

There are additional requirements for prescribing a Schedule-II substance. Most states require that these prescriptions be completed on a triplicate prescription. Many states allow written prescriptions for C-II drugs to be valid for only seven days, and these orders are prohibited from having authorized refills.

The dispensing of controlled substances is similar to that of legend drugs under the FDCA; however, there are several exceptions and additional regulations. In addition to the information required on the label for a noncontrolled legend prescription, controlled substances require a federal transfer warning; if the medication is a refill for a C-III or C-IV, the label must also include the date of initial filling, in addition to the date of the refill.

Ordering

To order Schedule I or Schedule II substances, a registrant must complete a triplicate form, the DEA form 222. However, registrants are not required to use the federal order form to obtain controlled substances in Schedule III, IV, or V due to their lower potential for abuse—in comparison to the other schedules.

Record Keeping

The CSA dictates that registrants keep records of the following items:

- "on-hand" inventory of controlled substances
- biennial inventory, after the initial inventory of controlled substances

There are additional records required, depending on the activity of the registrant.

The DEA requires exact quantities for Schedule I and II substances, while they permit an estimate quantity for Schedule III, IV, and V substances.

There are three approved filing methods for prescriptions of controlled substances:

1. Three Drawer—in which there is one file for C-II, one file for C-III, C-IV, C-V, and one file for all other prescriptions.

2. Two Drawer—in which there is one file for all controlled substances and one for all other prescriptions. Note that all prescriptions for Schedule III–V must have a red "C" stamped in the lower right corner.

3. Two Drawer—in which there is one drawer for C-II and one drawer for all other prescriptions, including Schedules III–V. Again, Schedules III–V must have a red "C" stamped in the lower right corner.

Reporting

If theft of controlled substances is discovered, the registrant must report the theft to both the DEA and the local police. The disposal of controlled substances must be reported to the DEA on DEA Form 41.

Inspections

The DEA may inspect any location registered for controlled substances. They may inspect all records, reports, forms, physical inventories, prescriptions, containers, labels, and equipment pertaining to controlled substances. They may also inspect security systems and/or take a physical inventory of all controlled substances.

OMNIBUS BUDGET RECONCILIATION ACT OF 1990

Known as OBRA '90, this act focused on the federal government funding of the Medicare and Medicaid programs. This was the act that mandated an increased necessity for pharmacy technicians. While determining the funding, OBRA also mandated that the pharmacist perform DUR (drug utilization reviews) and offer counseling to patients, and even provided funding and set fees for the reimbursement for such activities. Besides elevating the profession of the pharmacists in the United States, OBRA, by its nature, created a real need for pharmacy technicians to assist the pharmacist.

HIPAA

The Health Insurance Portability and Accountability Act of 1996 (HIPAA) focuses on patient confidentiality and privacy. Initially, HIPAA gave patients the right to review their medical records and established the requirement of patient consent for the transfer of medical records or oral, written, and electronic communications regarding medical records. Today, patient consent is required for a pharmacist or pharmacy technician to fill a prescription.

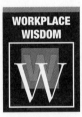

WORKPLACE WISDOM

As pharmacy technicians are assuming more responsibility and receiving greater roles and recognition in the pharmacy, they are also becoming more liable. Professional liability insurance coverage is now offered by a number of providers, including Pharmacists Mutual, based in Algona, Iowa.

HIPAA considers the following as protected health information (PHI):

- any information created or received by the pharmacy
- information relating to a patient's health—mental or physical, past, present, or future
- information that may identify a patient

CONCLUSION

In addition to the federal laws covered in this chapter, many of the regulations pertaining to practicing as a pharmacy technician are established and regulated by your specific state board of pharmacy. In general, federal laws pertain to the manufacturing of pharmaceutical products, and state laws pertain to the actual dispensing of those products. It is imperative that you familiarize yourself with both the federal laws and those pertaining to pharmacy practice in your particular state.

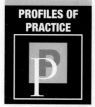

PROFILES OF PRACTICE

Disasters prompted the U.S. government to establish many of the original laws pertaining to pharmacy practice and the efficacy of medications. In 1937, a manufacturer decided to market a mixture of sulfanilamide and diethylene glycol as a remedy for sore throats. Diethylene glycol, however, is known today as antifreeze, and caused the mixture to be a deadly poison. This issue, which caused 107 reported deaths and became known as the Sulfanilamide Disaster of 1937, prompted the passing of the FDCA of 1938.

CHAPTER REVIEW QUESTIONS

1. The moral principle focusing on acting with self reliance is:
   - **a.** beneficence
   - **c.** veracity
   - **b.** fidelity
   - **d.** autonomy

2. The FDCA is administered by the:
   - **a.** FDA
   - **c.** NABP
   - **b.** DEA
   - **d.** CSA

3. Which one of the following requires that prescription drugs bear the legend "Caution: Federal law prohibits dispensing without a prescription" or "RX ONLY"?
   - **a.** Kefauver-Harris Amendments
   - **b.** Durham-Humphrey Amendment
   - **c.** HIPAA
   - **d.** OBRA '90

4. Thermometers are classified as:
   - **a.** Class I Devices
   - **c.** Class III Devices
   - **b.** Class II Devices
   - **d.** Class IV Devices

5. Which of the following established good manufacturing practices for drug manufacturers?
   - **a.** Kefauver-Harris Amendments
   - **b.** Durham-Humphrey Amendment
   - **c.** HIPAA
   - **d.** OBRA '90

6. Marijuana is classified as:
   - **a.** C-I   **b.** C-II   **c.** C-III   **d.** C-IV

7. A drug that is in a condition contrary to the intentions of the manufacturer is called:
   - **a.** a controlled substance
   - **b.** OTC
   - **c.** misbranded
   - **d.** adulterated

8. The CSA established ___ classes for controlled substances.
   - **a.** 5   **b.** 4   **c.** 3   **d.** 2

9. Schedule II drugs are permitted to have ___ refills.
   - **a.** 5   **b.** 1   **c.** 6   **d.** no

10. The form required to order C-II drugs is:
    - **a.** DEA 41
    - **c.** DEA 224
    - **b.** DEA 222
    - **d.** DEA 225

Resources and References

1. Buerki, Robert A. and Louis D. Vottero. *Ethical Practices in Pharmacy: A Guidebook for Pharmacy Technicians.* Madison, WI: American Institute of the History of Pharmacy, 1997.

2. Nielsen, James Robert. *Handbook of Federal Drug Law*, 2d ed. Baltimore, MD: Williams & Wilkins, 1992.

3. Porter, Vanessa. Pharmacy Law & Patient Confidentiality: *Today's Technician Magazine* Volume 3 Issue 4. Houston, TX: National Pharmacy Technician Association, 2003.

Terminology
and Abbreviations

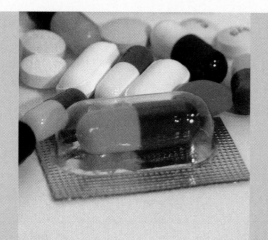

After completing this chapter, you
should be able to:

- Identify the basic root words
  used in everyday pharmacy
  settings.

- Identify the basic prefixes and
  suffixes used in various
  pharmacy settings.

- List the common abbreviations
  used by pharmacy and medical
  professionals.

- List the abbreviations written
  on a prescription for dispensing
  purposes.

INTRODUCTION

In order to understand the pharmacy industry and profession,
you must learn the appropriate language. The terminology in
this chapter comprises the most common words and phrases
as well as prefixes and suffixes used to communicate in the
practice of pharmacy. This chapter will give you an overview
of the standard terminology that you will need to know in
order to succeed. The information is arranged by topic, and
then alphabetically, for easier reference in the future. This
chapter is not all-inclusive; you should continue to learn as
much terminology as possible to better increase your
knowledge base.

Understanding Selected Roots

Root words are words or parts of a word that identify the major meaning of the word. Root words are the essential part of the whole word. More specifically, root words can identify what part of the body or condition a term relates to. By your ability to identify roots, prefixes, and suffixes, you will be able to understand words you have never seen or heard before. You will find some of the common root words used in various pharmacy settings in the following list:

arter—artery	my—muscle
arthr—joint	nasa—nose
bronch—bronchus	nephr—kidney
carcin—cancer	neur—nerve
cardi—heart	oste—bone
cutane—skin	phleb—vein
cyst—bladder	pneum—lung
derma—skin	pulmo—lung
enter—abdomen (intestine)	ren—kidney
gastro—stomach	rhine—nose
gluc—sugar	thromb—blood clot
hemat—blood	vas—blood vessel
hepat—liver	ven—vein
lipid—fat	

Understanding Selected Prefixes

A prefix is a part of a word attached to the beginning of the root word, giving a specific meaning to the root. Prefixes are commonly used in the medical field in order to recognize the meaning of a bigger word. Following are some of the common prefixes you will encounter as a pharmacy technician:

a, an—without	extra—outside, in addition
angio—blood or lymph vessel	gluc—glucose
ante—before	hyper—too much
anti—inhibit, oppose	hypo—too little
arterio—artery	hyper—high
bio—living organisms	hypo—low
brady—slow	inter—between, among
cide—kill	intra—within
cervic—neck	macro—large, long
contra—against	mal—abnormal
de—remove from	mega—large
dys—abnormal, difficult	micro—small
endo—inside	nephro—kidney

neo—new
osteo—bone
para—around
phag—eat
phleb—vein
poly—many, much
post—after, behind

pre—before, in front
psych—mind, mental
pulmo—lung
sub—below, underlying
tachy—too fast
vaso—blood vessels

Understanding Selected Suffixes

A suffix is a part of a word attached to the end of the root word, giving a specific, new meaning to the root word. The following are the more common suffixes a pharmacy technician should be familiar with and understand:

algia—painful
ase—enzyme
cide—kill, killer
ectomy—surgical removal
emia—blood condition
pnea—to breathe
facient —causing, making
ia—condition of
ism—condition, state of
itis—inflammation

logy—study of
oma—tumor, lump, swelling
osis—condition of
ostomy—surgical opening
pathy—disease
penia—deficiency
sclerosis—hardening
tension—pressure

Pharmacy Abbreviations

Similar to the medical field, the pharmacy setting is full of abbreviations, acronyms, and codes. In order to completely understand the language, you must understand and interpret these abbreviations. The abbreviations are not federally recognized, but favored as a standard meaning for the whole word or phrase. It is much easier to read a couple of symbols than to interpret a physician's poor handwriting. Symbols and abbreviations are also used as a time saving measure for the physician and pharmacy staff. In order to prepare a prescription for dispensing, you must be able to interpret the medication order as written by the physician. Following are the common abbreviations used when writing a prescription as well as those used for standard pharmacy practice:

PRESCRIPTION ABBREVIATIONS

Adverse drug effect—ADE
Adverse drug reaction—ADR
Average wholesale price—AWP
Compound—cmpd; cpd

Concentration—conc
Diagnosis related group—DRG
Discontinue—D/C; DC
Dispense—disp.

Dispense as written—DAW

Drug Enforcement Agency—DEA

Drug utilization review—DUR

Elixir—elix

Enteric coated—EC

Fluid—fl

Food and Drug Administration—FDA

Maximum allowable cost—MAC

No known allergies—NKA

Nothing by mouth—NPO

Occupational Safety and Health Association—OSHA

Over-the-counter—OTC

Pediatric—ped

Prescription—Rx

Schedule I—C-I

Schedule II—C-II

Schedule III—C-III

Schedule IV—C-IV

Schedule V—C-V

Solution—soln

Syrup—syr

Therapeutic equivalence evaluation code—TEE

Vitamin—vit

Water—aq, aqua

Wholesale acquisition cost—WAC

PRESCRIPTION DIRECTIONS (SIG. CODES)

After—p

After meals—pc

After meals and at bedtime—pc&hs

Afternoon—pm

As desired—ad lib

As directed—u.d.

Sufficient quantity—q.s.

As needed—prn

As soon as possible—ASAP

Bedtime—hs

Before meals—ac

Before meals and at bedtime—ac&hs

Both ears—AU

Both eyes—OU

By mouth—po; PO

Daily; once daily—qd; QD

Dispense as written—DAW

Double strength—DS

Every—q; Q

Everyday—qd; QD

Everyday at bedtime—qhs; QHS

Every afternoon/evening—qpm; QPM

Every hour—qh; QH

Every morning—qam; QAM

Every other day—qod; QOD

Every week—qw

Four times daily—qid; QID

Hour—hr

Left ear—AS

Left eye—OS

May repeat—MR

Normal saline—NS

Right ear—AD

Right eye—OD

Three times daily—tid; TID

Two times daily; twice daily—bid; BID

As directed—Ut. Dict.

Weekly—w, wk

With—c

Without—s

While awake—W/A; WA

24 hours—24H

ROUTES OF ADMINISTRATION

Buccal—BU

By mouth; orally—PO

External—EX

Inhalation—IN

Injection—IJ

Intradermal—ID

Intramuscular—IM

Intravenous—IV

Intravenous piggyback—IVPB

Intravenous push—IVP

Intrauterine—IU

Metered dose inhaler—MDI

Mouth/throat—MT

Nasal—NA

Ointment—oint; ung

Ophthalmic—oph; ophth

Oral—OR

Otic—OT

Rectally—PR; RE

Subcutaneous—SC

Sublingual—SL

Suppository—supp

Tincture—tinct.

Transdermal—TD

Urethral—UR

Vaginally—PV; VA

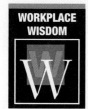

WORKPLACE WISDOM

You must be precise and cautious when using medical or pharmacy abbreviations—many are very similar, but have significantly different meanings.

MEASUREMENT ABBREVIATIONS

Ampule—amp

Capsule—cap

Centimeter—cm

Cubic centimeters—cc

Drop—gtt

Each—aa, ea

Fluid ounce—fl oz

Grain—gr.

Gram—g; gm

Hour—H; hr

Kilogram—kg

Liquid—liq

Liter—L

Microgram—mcg

Milligram—mg

Milliequivalent—mEq

Milliliter—ml

Millimeter—mm

One-half—ss

Ounce—oz

Pound—lb; #

Tablespoon—tbsp; TBS

Tablet—tab

Teaspoon—tsp

Units—u

MEDICAL ABBREVIATIONS

Acetaminophen—apap; APAP

Acquired immune deficiency syndrome—AIDS

Aspirin—asa; ASA

Attention deficit disorder—ADD

Attention deficit hyperactivity disorder—ADHD

Autonomic nervous system—ANS

Before surgery—pre op

Birth control pills—BCP; BC

Blood pressure—BP

Blood sugar—BS

Bowel movement—BM

Calcium—Ca

Carbohydrate—Carb

Central nervous system—CNS

Congestive heart failure—CHF

Discontinue—D/C; DC

Electrocardiogram—ECG; EKG

Electroencephalogram—EEG

Gastrointestinal—GI

Genitourinary—GU

Headache—HA

Health maintenance
organization—HMO

History—Hx

Human immunodeficiency
virus—HIV

Hydrochlorothiazide—HCTZ

Hydrogen peroxide—H_2O_2

Intensive care unit—ICU

Iron—Fe

Magnesium—Mg

Magnesium oxide—MgO;
MagOx

Managed care organization—
MCO

Milk of magnesia—MOM

Multiple vitamin—MV; MVI

Nausea and vomiting—N/V;
N&V

Nitroglycerine—NTG

Nonsedating antihistamines—
NSAs

Nonsteroidal anti-inflammatory
drugs—NSAIDs

Penicillin—PCN

Potassium—K

Potassium chloride—KCl

Preferred provider
organization—PPO

Sodium—Na

Sodium chloride—NaCl

Tetracycline—TCN

Urinary tract infection—UTI

Dangerous Abbreviations

It is important to note that, effective January 1, 2004, a list of dangerous abbreviations, acronyms, and symbols not to be used, known as the "Do Not Use" list, was issued by the Joint Commission on the Accreditation of Healthcare Organizations (JCAHO). One of the major problems with certain abbreviations is that they may have more than one meaning. For example, "DC" could mean Discharge in one instance or Discontinue in another; or, poorly written, "QD" could look more like "QID" to someone else.

With communication of medical records and documentation spanning across various health care venues, abbreviations increase the percentage of risk for misinterpretation. In addition, some health care staff may be unfamiliar with certain abbreviations, which can cause a delay in health care to the patient. The primary benefit of the exclusion of dangerous abbreviations is patient safety.

The following items are affected by this initiative:

- medication orders
- clinical documentation
- progress notes
- consultation reports
- operative reports
- educational materials

- protocols
- other related

The Institute of Medicine (IOM) issued a report in 1999 which stated that between 44,000 and 96,000 deaths each year may be attributed to medical errors. In light of this information, numerous health care entities are continuously evaluating and developing strategies for reducing these large numbers. One result has been the development of the "Do Not Use" list, which is based on the most commonly mistaken and misunderstood written abbreviations used in all forms of medical communication. As of January 1, 2004, a "minimum" list of dangerous abbreviations, acronyms, and symbols has been approved by JCAHO. (See Table 3-1.)

Beginning January 1, 2004, the following items *must* be included on each accredited organization's "Do not use" list (Table 3-1):

TABLE 3-1 "Minimum List" of Dangerous Abbreviations, Acronyms, and Symbols*

Abbreviation	Potential Problem	Preferred Term
U (for unit)	Mistaken as zero, four, or cc.	Write "unit"
IU (for international unit)	Mistaken as IV (intravenous) or 10 (ten)	Write "international unit"
Q.D., Q.O.D. (Latin abbreviation for once daily and every other day)	Mistaken for each other. The period after the Q can be mistaken for an "I" and the "O" can be mistaken for "I"	Write "daily" and "every other day"
Trailing zero (X.0 mg), Lack of leading zero (.X mg)	Decimal point is missed	Never write a zero by itself after a decimal point (X mg), and always use a zero before a decimal point (0.X mg)
MS MSO$_4$ MgSO$_4$	Confused for one another. Can mean morphine sulfate or magnesium sulfate	Write "morphine sulfate" or "magnesium sulfate"

* http://www.aapmr.org/hpl/pracguide/jcahosymbols.htm

In addition to these basic mandatory items that should no longer be used, as of April 1, 2004, each organization must identify and apply at least three additional "Do not use" abbreviations, acronyms, or symbols of its own choosing. Table 3-2 offers suggestions for items that should be considered for each facility's "Do not use " list.

In addition, the Institute for Safe Medical Practices (ISMP), has suggested other abbreviations, acronyms, and symbols that should be taken into consideration. Optimally, all these terms should be prohibited also. (See Table 3-3.)

Further details are available on the following JCAHO and ISMP websites:

- *www.jcaho.com*
- *www.ISMP.org*

TABLE 3-2 Suggested Items in Addition to the "Minimum Required List"*

Abbreviation	Potential Problem	Preferred Term
μg (for microgram)	Mistaken for mg (milligrams) resulting in one thousand-fold dosing overdose.	Write "mcg."
H.S. (for half-strength or Latin abbreviation for bedtime)	Mistaken for either half-strength or hour of sleep (at bedtime). q.H.S. mistaken for every hour. All can result in a dosing error.	Write out "half-strength" or "at bedtime."
T.I.W. (for three times a week)	Mistaken for three times a day or twice weekly, resulting in an overdose.	Write "3 times weekly" or "three times weekly."
S.C. or S.Q. (for subcutaneous)	Mistaken as SL for sublingual, or "5 every."	Write "Sub-Q," "subQ," or "subcutaneously."
D/C (for discharge)	Interpreted as discontinue whatever medications follow (typically discharge meds).	Write "discharge."
c.c. (for cubic centimeter)	Mistaken for U (units) when poorly written.	Write "ml" for milliliters.
A.S., A.D., A.U. (Latin abbreviation for left, right, or both ears) O.S., O.D., O.U. (Latin abbreviation for left, right, or both eyes)	Mistaken for each other (e.g., AS for OS, AD for OD, AU for OU, etc.).	Write: "left ear," "right ear," or "both ears"; "left eye," "right eye," or "both eyes."

http://www.aapmr.org/hpl/pracguide/jcahosymbols.htm

TABLE 3-3 Special Issue—Do not use the following dangerous abbreviations or dose designations:

Abbreviation/Dose Expression	Intended Meaning	Misinterpretation	Correction
Apothecary symbols	*dram* *minim*	*Misunderstood or misread (symbol for dram misread for "3" and minim misread as "mL").*	*Use the metric system.*
AU	aurio uterque (each ear)	Mistaken for OU (oculo uterque—each eye).	Don't use this abbreviation.
D/C	discharge discontinue	Premature discontinuation of medications when D/C (intended to mean "discharge") has been misinterpreted as "discontinued" when followed by a list of drugs.	Use "discharge" and "discontinue."

Drug names			Use the complete spelling for drug names.
ARA^{o}A	vidarabine	cytarabineARA^{o}C	
AZT	zidovudine (Retrovir)	azathioprine	
CPZ	Compazine (prochlorperazine)	chlorpromazine	
DPT	Demerol-Phenergan-Thorazine	diphtheria-pertussis-tetanus (vaccine)	
HCl	hydrochloric acid	potassium chloride (The "H" is misinterpreted as "K.")	
HCT	hydrocortisone	hydrochlorothiazide	
HCTZ	hydrochlorothiazide	hydrocortisone (seen as HCT250 mg)	
MgSO$_4$	magnesium sulfate	morphine sulfate	
MSO$_4$	morphine sulfate	magnesium sulfate	
MTX	methotrexate	mitoxantrone	
TAC	triamcinolone	tetracaine, Adrenalin, cocaine	
ZnSO$_4$	zinc sulfate	morphine sulfate	

Stemmed names			
"Nitro" drip	nitroglycerin infusion	sodium nitroprusside infusion	
"Norflox"	norfloxacin	Norflex	
m g	microgram	Mistaken for "mg" when handwritten.	Use "mcg."
o.d. or OD	once daily	Misinterpreted as "right eye" (OD—oculus dexter) and administration of oral medications in the eye.	Use "daily."
TIW or tiw	three times a week.	Mistaken as "three times a day."	Don't use this abbreviation.
per os	orally	The "os" can be mistaken for "left eye."	Use "PO," "by mouth," or "orally."
q.d. or QD	every day	Mistaken as q.i.d., especially if the period after the "q" or the tail of the "q" is read as an "i."	Use "daily" or "every day."
qn	nightly or at bedtime	Misinterpreted as "qh" (every hour).	Use "nightly."
qhs	nightly at bedtime	Misread as every hour.	Use "nightly."
q6PM, etc.	every evening at 6 p.m.	Misread as every six hours.	Use 6 p.m. "nightly."

Abbreviation/Dose Expression	Intended Meaning	Misinterpretation	Correction
q.o.d. or QOD	every other day	Misinterpreted as "q.d." (daily) or "q.i.d. (four times daily) if the "o" is poorly written.	Use "every other day."
sub q	subcutaneous	The "q" has been mistaken for "every" (e.g., one heparin dose ordered "sub q 2 hours before surgery" misinterpreted as every two hours before surgery).	Use "subcut." or write "subcutaneous."
SC	subcutaneous	Mistaken for SL (sublingual).	Use "subcut." or write "subcutaneous."
U or u	unit	Read as a zero (0) or a four (4), causing a 10 fold overdose or greater (4U seen as "40" or 4u seen as "44").	"Unit" has no acceptable abbreviation. Use "unit."
IU	international unit	Misread as IV (intravenous).	Use "units."
cc	cubic centimeters	Misread as "U" (units).	Use "mL."
x3d	for three days	Mistaken for "three doses."	Use "for three days."
BT	bedtime	Mistaken as "BID" (twice daily).	Use "hs."
ss	sliding scale (insulin) or $\frac{1}{2}$ (apothecary)	Mistaken for "55."	Spell out "sliding scale." Use "one-half" or use "$\frac{1}{2}$."
> and <	greater than and less than	Mistakenly used for the opposite of intended meaning.	Use "greater than" or "less than."
/ (slash mark)	separates two doses or indicates "per"	Misunderstood as the number 1 ("25 unit/10 units" read as "110" units.	Do not use a slash mark to separate elements in doses. Use "per."
Name letters and dose numbers run together (e.g., Inderal40 mg)	Inderal 40 mg	Misread as Inderal 140 mg.	Always use space between drug name, dose, and unit of measure.
Zero after decimal point (1.0)	1 mg	Misread as 10 mg if the decimal point is not seen.	Do not use terminal zeros for doses expressed in whole numbers.
No zero before decimal dose (.5 mg)	0.5 mg	Misread as 5 mg.	Always use zero before a decimal when the dose is less than a whole unit.

Terminology

Terminology is the set of technical or special terms used in a business, art, science, or specific profession. Like many professions, pharmacy and medical professionals use a unique language and terminology. The following lists are not complete, but are a good reference when working in a pharmacy.

PHARMACEUTICAL TERMINOLOGY

A

Absorption is the time it takes for a drug to work after the drug has been administered; the rate at which the drug passes from the intestines into the bloodstream.

Acute refers to a disease or illness with a sudden onset and a short duration.

Active ingredient is the chemical found in the medication known or believed to have a therapeutic effect.

Additive is a substance added to a liquid solution intended for IV use.

Admixture is a substance produced by mixing two or more substances.

Adverse reaction denotes an unwanted or unexpected side effect or reaction to a medication; it may also result from an interaction among two or more medications.

Aerosol is a medication dosage form that contains a gaseous substance consisting of fine liquid or solid particles.

Alcoholic solution is a solution that contains only alcohol as the dissolving agent.

Allergic reaction denotes a sensitivity to a specific substance that is absorbed through the skin, inhaled into the lungs, swallowed, or injected.

Allergy is a sensitivity of the immune system to a chemical or drug; an allergy causes symptoms ranging from rashes to more severe symptoms such as irregular breathing.

Amphetamines are substances that are frequently abused as a stimulant medication; they can be used to treat the medical conditions of narcolepsy and eating disorders.

Analgesic refers to a substance used to relieve acute or chronic pain.

Analeptic refers to a substance that stimulates the central nervous system.

Anaphylactic shock is a hypersensitivity reaction to a substance.

Anesthetic refers to relief of pain by the process of interfering with the nerve transmission alerting the brain of pain.

Angiotensin-converting enzyme (ACE) inhibitors are used to treat hypertension (high blood pressure) and heart failure by blocking the enzyme that activates angiotensin—a natural substance that narrows the blood vessels causing high blood pressure.

Anorectic refers to a substance that suppresses the appetite.

Antacid is a substance that relieves high acid levels in the gastric (stomach) area.

Antagonist refers to a substance that opposes the action of another drug or substance.

Antianxiety describes substances that reduce or relieve anxiety.

Antibiotic is a substance that is used to kill or stop the growth of bacteria in the body.

Antibody is a protein produced by the immune system to respond to foreign substances in the body.

Anticholinergic refers to a substance that inhibits hypersecretion and GI motility.

Anticoagulant refers to a substance that stops blood clotting (also known as a blood thinner).

Anticonvulsant refers to a substance that stops brain nerve firing to suppress convulsive seizures.

Antidepressant is a substance that helps to maintain proper hormone balance levels to decrease depressive moods.

Antidiarrheal relieves and decreases GI activity that produces diarrhea.

Antidote is a substance or remedy that counteracts the effects of a poisoning agent.

Antiemetic relieves nausea and vomiting.

Antiflatulent refers to a substance that relieves the pressure of excess intestinal gas.

Antifungal refers to a substance that kills fungus growing in the body.

Antihistamine refers to a substance that stops the effects of histamine release that causes sneezing, watery eyes, and congestion.

Antihypertensive substances work to lower blood pressure.

Antiinflammatory substances reduce and relieve inflammation.

Antineoplastic substances are used to kill cancer cells.

Antioxidant is a chemical substance produced by the body in response to a foreign organism, bacteria, or virus.

Antiplatelets are substances that reduce the ability of platelets to stick together and form a clot.

Antipruritic denotes a substance that relieves itching.

Antipyretic refers to a substance that relieves and lowers high fever.

Antipsychotics are substances that block and inhibit the stimulatory actions of dopamine.

Antispasmodics relieve stomach muscle spasms.

Antitussives relieve severe cough.

Antiviral refers to drugs that fight viral infections in the body.

Aqueous means "containing water."

Aseptic techniques are used to get rid of and protect against bacteria and other microorganisms.

Astringent refers to a substance that stops secretions or controls bleeding.

Auxiliary labels are placed on the medication package to provide information and instructions for use.

B

Beta-blockers are substances used in the treatment of hypertension, angina, arrhythmia, and cardiomyopathy; they may also be used to minimize the possibility of sudden death after a heart attack.

Binding agent is a substance that holds all of the ingredients in a tablet together.

Bioequivalence describes a substance acting on the body with the same strength and similar bioavailability as the same dosage of a sample of a given substance.

Blood sugar level is the measure of glucose (sugar) level in the bloodstream.

Brand name is the proprietary name of a drug exclusive to a manufacturer for selling and distributing purposes.

Bronchodilator is a substance that relaxes the bronchial smooth muscles in the respiratory system.

Buccal tablet is a tablet that is dissolved in the lining of the cheek instead of being swallowed whole.

Bulk compounding is the process of compounding large quantities of a substance for dispensing or distributing.

Bulk manufacturing is the process of manufacturing large quantities of a substance for sales and distribution.

Bulking agent is a chemical substance required in order to produce a certain desired result.

C

Calcium-channel blockers are substances used to treat and reduce hypertension (high blood pressure) and disorders that affect the blood supply to the heart; also used in the treatment of irregular heartbeats.

Capsule is a solid dosage form of a medication usually made of gelatin, which holds fine particles of a solid or liquid particle.

Chewable tablets are chewed instead of swallowed whole.

Chronic refers to a disease or illness that has a long duration (i.e., lifetime).

Clinical trials are scientific experiments that test the effect of a drug in human test patients; required by the FDA for approval of a new medication.

Communicable refers to a disease or illness that can be transmitted to another person.

Compound refers to substance made from a combination of two or more substances.

Contagious refers to the time period when an infectious person can transmit a disease to another person through direct or indirect contact.

Contraindication is an aspect of a patient's condition that does not agree with the treatment.

Controlled released medications are released and metabolized over a period of time in the body.

Controlled substance refers to a drug with a high abuse potential; the manufacturing and distribution are regulated by the federal government to limit abuse and harm.

Corticosteroids are substances used to prevent minor asthma attacks or to treat severe attacks.

Cream is a dosage form of a medication that is a semisolid preparation, usually applied externally to soothe, lubricate, or protect.

Cure is the effective treatment of a disease or illness leading to elimination of all symptoms.

D

Decongestant refers to a substance that shrinks the mucous membranes that produce congestion.

Dehydration refers to excessive loss of water from the body.

Diagnosis is a process by which a health care professional (doctor, nurse, or technician) determines the patient's condition or disease, following tests and examinations.

Disease is a physical process in which the body or specific organs are being destroyed, causing harm and characteristic symptoms to the patient.

Distribution is the process following absorption by which a drug is passed to the cells of various organs.

Diuretic is a substance that increases the water output in the kidneys; reduces water retention in the body.

Dopamine is a neurotransmitter associated with the regulation of movement, emotions, pain, and pleasure.

Drops are a liquid dosage form of medication that are placed in the eye or ear.

Drug is a chemical compound intended for the use in diagnosis, treatment, or prevention of a disease in human or animals; any substance that is intended to produce an alteration of the chemistry and/or functioning of the body.

E

Effervescent tablet is a tablet that is dissolved into a liquid before administration.

Electrolytes are salts that the body requires in its fluids that are essential in nerve, muscle, and heart functions.

Elimination is the process following distribution by which the drug is broken down and the excess is excreted through urine.

Elixir is a liquid dosage form that contains flavored water and alcohol mixtures.

Emulsion is a liquid dosage form of a mixture of two products that normally do not mix together.

Enema is the process by which a medicated fluid is injected into the rectum.

Esophagitis is a condition characterized by inflammation, swelling, and irritation of the esophagus.

Estrogens are hormones that are produced in the ovaries and are responsible for the development and maintenance of female secondary sex characteristics.

Excretion is the process by which the body eliminates waste after metabolism and distribution.

Expectorants are substances that remove mucous from the upper respiratory system.

F

Food and Drug Administration (FDA) is the federal agency responsible for the approval, review, and regulation of drugs and dietary supplements.

Formulary refers to a list of preferred medications that insurance plans allow the members to get at a lower out-of-pocket expense.

Fungicide refers to a substance that kills fungi.

G

Generic name is the nonproprietary name of a drug.

Genetically engineered drugs are substances that have had foreign genes artificially inserted into their genetic codes.

Glucagon is a hormone produced in the pancreas that causes the automatic release of glucose.

Glucose is the primary energy source and sugar found in the bloodstream.

Glycogen is the principal substance the body uses for storing carbohydrates; stored in the liver, turns into glucose and releases into the bloodstream when the blood sugar level gets low.

H

Half-life defines the amount of time it takes for half of a substance to be broken down in the body and excreted.

Hazardous waste is any substance that is potentially dangerous and toxic to living organisms; must be disposed of properly.

Health is the physical, emotional, or mental well-being of a person.

Health care procedures, techniques, tests, and examinations are used to prevent, treat, and maintain a patient's health and well-being.

Histamine (H2) blockers reduce acid secretion by blocking histamine from reaching the H2 receptors.

Hydroalcoholic solution contains water and alcohol.

Hypersensitivity is an exaggerated response to a given stimulus.

Hypnotic refers to a substance that relaxes the central nervous system to produce sleep.

I

Immediate released medications are released and metabolized immediately following administration.

Immunosuppressant refers to substances that are used to prevent the body from rejecting an organ transplant (also known as anti-rejection drugs).

Inactive ingredients are the remaining ingredients, other than the active ingredient, that are found in a drug; used to flavor, digest, color, and bind the whole substance.

Infusion is the process of a slow injection of solution or emulsion into a vein or subcutaneous tissue.

Inhalation is the administration of a medication directly into the lungs by the mouth or nose.

Inhaler is a dosage form that uses a gaseous substance to force fine solid or liquid particles into the respiratory system through the nose or mouth.

Insulin is a hormone secreted by the pancreas that helps the body to digest sugars and starches; manufactured insulin is available for use when the pancreas does not produce enough on its own.

Intolerance is an extreme sensitivity to a drug or other substance.

Intracardiac denotes the administration of a medication by injection directly into the heart.

Intradermal denotes the administration of a medication by injection into the skin.

Intramuscular refers to the administration of a medication within or into a muscle(s).

Intravenous refers to the administration of a medication within or into a vein(s).

Inventory refers to the supplies of medications that the pharmacy stocks for dispensing.

L

Labeling is the process of identifying a particular medication with the patient's and physician's information for dispensing.

Laxative is a substance that increases defecation.

Legend drug is a medication that requires a prescription written by a physician before it can be dispensed to the patient.

Local refers to a small area or single part of the body (e.g., local anesthetic).

Lotion is a liquid dosage form that contains a powdered substance in a suspension, used externally to soothe, cool, dry, and protect.

M

Medical devices are devices or products used for medical procedures or diagnostic tests.

Medication order is a prescription usually given in a hospital or other institutional setting.

Migraines are severe headache caused by extreme changes in the blood vessels in the brain.

Muscle relaxants are used to treat involuntary, painful contraction of muscles by slowing the passages of nerve signals that cause pain to the muscles.

N

Narcotic is a drug that is potentially highly abused as a pain reliever, causing dependency and tolerance.

Narrow therapeutic range is the bioequivalence range of a brand drug and its generic counterpart where very small changes in dosage level could result in toxicity.

Nonaqueous means "contains no water."

Nonlegend drugs are medications that do not require a prescription before dispensing; more commonly referred to as over-the-counter medications.

Nonsteroidal anti-inflammatory agents are substances that inhibit the production of the enzymes necessary for the synthesis of prostaglandins, reducing pain and inflammation.

O

Ointment is a semisolid (mixture of a liquid and solid) dosage form that is applied externally to deliver medication, lubricate, and protect.

Ophthalmic refers to administration of a medication through the eye.

Opiate is a drug that originates from the opium poppy, such as morphine or codeine.

Opioid is a drug, hormone, or other substance that has sedative or narcotic effects similar to substances containing opium or its derivatives.

Oral refers to the administration of a medication into the mouth.

OSHA—Occupational Health and Safety Association—is responsible for safety guidelines in the workplace.

Otic denotes the administration of a medication into the ear.

Overdose is the action of, and condition resulting from, ingesting too much of a substance or drug; may result from one dose, or multiple doses over the course of time.

P

Package insert is a supplement provided by the manufacturer regarding specific details, instructions, and warnings about the medication.

Parenteral denotes the administration of medication by any other route than oral; administration by injection.

Patch is a dosage form in which the medication is delivered through a solid application applied to the skin and absorbed into the bloodstream.

Patent is a federally granted, exclusive right to a product for a specific period of time (before other manufacturers can create and sell the identical product).

Pharmacist is a licensed health care professional skilled and trained to dispense medications as ordered by a physician and to counsel patients on their drug therapies.

Pharmacokinetics is the study of the rates at which drugs are metabolized, distributed, and excreted from the body after consumption.

Pharmacology is the study of drugs and their effects on the body.

Placebo is a pill-like preparation that contains no active or chemical ingredient, usually given for its psychological effects (commonly referred to as a sugar pill).

Prescription includes a direction given by a physician for the preparation and use of a medication for a specific patient, to be dispensed by a pharmacist.

Progestins are female reproductive hormones; they cause menstruation as they trigger the shedding of the uterine lining.

Proton pump inhibitors are substances that reduce gastric acid build-up by blocking the release of protons by proton pumps.

Psychotherapeutic drugs are substances used to relieve the symptoms of mental and psychiatric illnesses, such as depression, psychosis, and anxiety.

Psychotropic denotes a substance that affects a person's ability to distinguish reality from the imaginary.

R

Recreational drugs (usually illegal) are often used in a social setting for their pleasurable effects instead of for their medicinal value.

Rectally refers to the administration of a solid or liquid medication given through the rectum.

S

Schedule I drugs are classified by the Drug Enforcement Agency as having a high abuse potential, with no FDA approval for medicinal use (illegal drugs).

Schedule II drugs are classified by the Drug Enforcement Agency as having a high abuse potential, with severe dependence liability (e.g., narcotics, amphetamines, stimulants).

Schedule III drugs are classified by the Drug Enforcement Agency as having less abuse potential than Schedule II drugs and moderate dependence liability (e.g., nonnarcotic stimulants, nonbarbituate sedatives, anabolic steroids).

Schedule IV drugs are classified by the Drug Enforcement Agency as having less abuse potential than schedule III drugs and limited dependence liability (e.g., sedatives, antianxiety agents, nonnarcotic analgesics).

Schedule V drugs have limited abuse potential; they are available as prescription or over-the-counter drugs (e.g., cough syrups with small amounts of codeine, antitussives, antidiarrheals).

Sedative relieves anxiety and tension; calms and relaxes.

Side effects are predicted, unwanted reactions to a substance or combination of substances.

Slow release medications are released and metabolized over a period of time in the body.

Solution is a liquid dosage form in which the medication is completely dissolved in a liquid.

Sterilize means to cleanse objects, wounds, burns, and so on, of microorganisms, such as bacteria.

Stimulants are a class of medications that are intended to increase alertness and physical activity.

Subcutaneous refers to the administration of a medication given under the skin.

Sublingual tablet is a tablet that is dissolved under the tongue instead of being swallowed whole.

Suppository denotes the administration through the vagina or rectum of a solid medication (also called a suppository).

Suspension is a liquid dosage form in which the solid particles are not completely dissolved.

Symptom is a condition that usually comes before the onset of a disease or illness; an abnormality that provides evidence of the existence of a disease or illness.

Syrup is a liquid dosage form that consists of water and sugar mixed with the medication.

T

Tablet is a solid dosage form in which the ingredients are compacted into a small, formed shape.

Tolerance is the condition in which the body has become unresponsive to a substance after prolonged exposure.

Topical refers to a substance used externally for relief of swelling, itching, or infection.

Transdermal refers to administration of a medication through the skin (e.g., patches).

U

U.S. Pharmacopoeia (USP) is a nonprofit organization, recognized by the FDA, that publishes standards on prescription drugs, over-the-counter medications, dietary supplements, and health care products.

V

Vaginal tablet is a tablet that is dissolved in the mucous lining of the vagina.

Vaginally denotes the administration of a solid or liquid medication through the vagina.

Vasodilator is a substance that causes the blood vessels to widen.

W

Withdrawal symptom is an effect that can occur as the result of suddenly stopping the use of a substance after prolonged use.

MEDICAL TERMINOLOGY

A

Acne vulgaris is a skin condition that occurs due to the overproduction of oil by the oil glands of the skin and results in pimples, blackheads, and whiteheads on the surface of skin.

Addiction is the physical or psychological dependence on a chemical substance such as alcohol; any habit that cannot easily be given up.

Anatomy is the study of the structures in living things.

Amnesia is the loss of memory (may be short- or long-term).

Anemia is a condition in which the bloodstream has very few red blood cells that can carry oxygen to the tissues.

Anesthesiologists are physicians who specialize in administering drugs to anesthetize or sedate patients before surgical procedures; they monitor a patient's vital signs while the patient is under anesthesia.

Angina pectoris is a condition characterized by the attack of chest pain caused by an insufficient supply of oxygen to the heart.

Anorexia is an eating disorder characterized by a refusal to maintain body weight at a healthy range, low self-esteem, and an intense fear of gaining weight.

Arrhythmia is an irregular heartbeat.

Arteriosclerosis is a condition characterized by thickening and hardening of the arteries.

Arthritis is a condition characterized by inflammation of the joints.

Asthma is a condition that affects a patient's breathing by restricting the airways and oxygen supply due to inflammation, swelling, and irritation.

Attention deficit disorder (ADD) is a mental disorder characterized by developmentally inappropriate levels of attention, concentration, activity, distractibility, and impulsivity.

Attention deficit hyperactivity disorder (ADHD) is a mental disorder characterized by constant impulsive behavior, difficulty in concentration, and hyperactivity that decreases social, academic, or occupational functioning.

Autoimmune disorders are characterized by an immune response against the body's own tissues.

B

Bacteria refers to single-celled microorganisms that are abundant in most living things; may be beneficial or harmful to a person.

Benign refers to a condition or abnormal growth that is not cancerous (e.g., tumor, cyst).

Blood pressure measures the force exerted by blood against the walls of the arteries; measured when the heart contracts and relaxes.

Bloodstream is the area in which the blood flows through the capillaries, veins, and arteries.

Body mass index (BMI) is the measurement of body fat relative to the patient's height and weight.

Bronchitis is a medical condition characterized by an acute inflammation of the bronchial tubes in the lungs.

C

Carcinogen is any agent capable of causing cancer.

Cardiologists are physicians who are specialized in the treatment of cardiac (heart) disorders and illnesses.

Cardiovascular disease refers to conditions of the heart and circulation system.

Catalyst is a substance that speeds up a chemical reaction.

Cavity is a hollow space in a structure.

Cerebral refers to the brain.

Chemotherapy is the prevention or treatment of cancerous disease by the use of toxic chemical agents.

Cholesterol is a substance produced in the liver and used for normal body functions including production of hormones, bile, and vitamin D.

Clinical refers to diagnostic tests, labs, and procedures that require close observation of patients.

Congestive heart failure is a potentially fatal condition of the cardiovascular system wherein the heart has lost its ability to pump blood in and out.

Contraceptives are drugs or devices used for the prevention of pregnancy; can also be used for hormone regulation.

Cranial refers to the skull or head.

Cystitis is a condition of inflammation of the urinary bladder.

D

Dermatologists are physicians who specialize in the treatment of skin disorders and illnesses.

Dependency is the physical and/or psychological reliance on a habit or chemical substance.

Detoxification is the process by which the patient is medically supervised for the withdrawal of alcohol or drug dependency.

Dementia is a disease characterized by progressive memory loss as well as learning and thinking disorders; often leads to Alzheimer's disease.

Depression is a mental disorder wherein the person feels sad and helpless; characterized by personality changes and a loss of socialization, communication, and energy.

Diabetes is a condition characterized by the failure of the body to produce insulin, which is essential for digestion and for retrieving energy from food, in the pancreas.

Distal refers to the part that is farthest from the point of attachment.

E

Edema refers to the abnormal swelling of the body, caused by an increased build-up of fluids in tissues and organs.

Emergency medicine specialists are physicians who specialize in the treatment of emergency situations and trauma.

Emphysema is an irreversible disease (characterized by long-term smoking) in which there has been severe damage to the alveoli (tiny air sacs) in the lungs, resulting in a decrease in the exchange of gases; symptoms are wheezing, coughing, shortness of breath, and difficulty in breathing.

Endorphin is a chemical or ingredient produced by the body that relieves pain and stress.

Erythrocyte is a red blood cell.

Esophagitis is an inflammation of the esophagus due to acid build-up.

Euphoria is a feeling of great happiness and well-being.

Excretion is the process by which waste is eliminated from the body.

External refers to the outer or outside part of a structure.

G

Gastric ulcer is a tear in the normal tissue lining of the stomach wall.

Gastritis is an inflammation of the normal tissue lining of the stomach wall.

Gastroesophageal reflux disease (GERD) is a condition that occurs when food not completely digested is forced back up the esophagus; the food is very acidic and irritates the esophagus, causing heartburn and other symptoms.

Gastroenterologists are physicians who specialize in the treatment of digestive disorders and illnesses.

Gastrointestinal tract is the part of the digestive system that includes the mouth, esophagus, stomach, and intestines; aids in digesting and processing food in the body.

Geriatrics is the treatment of elderly patients.

Glaucoma is an eye condition caused by a build-up of pressure due to reduced drainage of fluid from the eye, possibly resulting in the loss of vision in that eye.

Gynecologists are physicians who specialize in the treatment of disorders of women's reproductive organs.

H

Heartburn is a painful burning sensation in the throat (esophagus) just below the breastbone.

Hemorrhage refers to severe, uncontrollable bleeding (can be external or internal).

Hepatitis is a condition associated with the inflammation of the liver.

Herpes simplex is an acute viral disease characterized by watery blisters on the skin and mucous membranes; commonly known as cold sores.

Hormone is a chemical substance that stimulates and regulates certain bodily functions.

Hormone Replacement Therapy (HRT) is a therapy developed for women to help increase the levels of estrogen that are declining during menopause.

Hyperglycemia is the condition of high blood glucose (sugar).

Hyperlipidemia refers to high cholesterol.

Hypertension refers to long-term high blood pressure.

Hypoglycemia is the condition of low blood glucose (sugar).

I

Immunity is the body's ability to fight off infections from bacteria and viruses.

Impotence is a condition characterized by the inability to achieve and maintain penile erection.

Inflammation is any redness, swelling, pain, or heat in a body tissue(s) caused by physical injury, infection, or irritation.

Influenza is a contagious viral infection of the nose, throat, and lungs, which often occurs in the winter season; also called "flu."

Inpatient refers to a person who has been admitted to a hospital or other medical facility to receive treatment for a disease.

Internal denotes the inner or inside part of a structure.

L

Leukemia is a condition characterized by elevated white blood cell counts.

Leukocyte is a white blood cell.

Lipids are organic compounds consisting of fats and other substances; used to measure cholesterol.

M

Malignant refers to an abnormal condition or growth in which a group of cells cause harm and destruction to other cells and tissues (e.g., cancerous cells).

Metastasis is the spreading of a disease from one organ or part of the body to another organ or part of the body.

Metabolism is defined as the physical and chemical processes of the body that convert consumed food into energy for use by the tissues and organs.

N

Narcolepsy is a rare, chronic sleep disorder characterized by constant daytime fatigue and sudden attacks of sleep.

Nausea is a feeling of sickness to the stomach, usually accompanied by the urge to vomit.

Neurologists are physicians who specialize in the treatment of disorders and illnesses within the brain and central nervous system.

Neuropathic relates to a disease of the nerves.

Neurotransmitter is a chemical substance released by one nerve cell that activates or inhibits a neighboring nerve cell.

O

Obstetricians are physicians who specialize in the care of pregnant women before and during the birth of babies.

Oncologists are physicians who specialize in the treatment of cancer and radiation therapy.

Ophthalmologists are physicians who specialize in the treatment of poor vision and eye disorders, using medication, corrective lenses, and surgery.

Organ is a part of the body made up of tissues and performs a specialized function; part of an organ system.

Orthopedists are physicians who specialize in the treatment of injuries and structural disorders of the bones and joints.

Osteoporosis is a medical disease characterized by a loss in total bone density; it can be the result of calcium deficiency, menopause, certain endocrine diseases, advanced age, medications, or other risk factors.

Otolaryngologists are physicians who specialize in the treatment of disorders and illnesses of the ear, nose, and throat.

Outpatient refers to patients who receive treatment from a hospital or other medical facility on a scheduled basis without being admitted for overnight or continuous stay.

P

Pain is a feeling of slight or severe discomfort caused by an injury or illness.

Panic attack is a sudden, repeated episode of extreme fear, panic, and anxiety.

Parietal refers to the wall of a structure.

Pathogen is a microorganism (bacteria or virus) that causes disease.

Pathologists study the history, causes, and progress of diseases by examining specimens of body tissues, blood, fluids, and secretions.

Pathology is the study of the nature of disease(s).

Peripheral denotes a location at or toward the surface of the body or its parts.

Physiology is the study of the function of living things.

Prevention is the process of taking steps beforehand to prevent a health condition or other abnormality from occurring or worsening.

Primary care is the medical care a person receives from a general practitioner or family physician.

Primary care physician is usually the internal medicine or family physician who is able to treat a variety of illnesses; refers a patient to a specialist if further specialized care or treatment is necessary.

Prognosis refers to the medical assessment of the expected outcome and course of a particular disease.

Proximal denotes the location of the part that is nearest to the point of attachment.

Psychiatrists are physicians who specialize in the treatment of mental, emotional, and behavioral disorders by the use of medications and psychotherapy.

Psychotherapy is the nondrug treatment of psychological disorders, usually performed as behavioral or cognitive therapy.

Pulmonary refers to the lungs and respiratory system.

R

Radiologists are technicians who use technologies such as X-rays, radiation therapy, and ultrasound machines to view and assess medical problems.

Receptor is the part of the nerve cell that recognizes the neurotransmitter and communicates with the other nerve cells.

Respiration is the process by which gases are passed through the lungs and distributed throughout the body.

S

Seasonal affective disorder (SAD) is a type of depression that occurs during the fall and winter months, or during other times of the year or in parts of the world where exposure to natural sunlight is limited.

Secondary care is medical care that a person receives from a specialist after being referred by his primary physician.

Serotonin is a neurotransmitter in the brain that functions to regulate moods, appetite, sensory perception, and other central nervous system functions.

Spasm is an involuntary muscle contraction.

Specialists are physicians who are experienced in a certain area of study for treatment and prevention.

Surgeons are physicians who are specialized in and trained to perform surgical procedures and operations on patients in order to provide treatment or cure for an illness or injury.

Syndrome refers to a set of symptoms that are characteristic of a particular disease.

Systemic refers to the whole body.

T

Terminally ill refers to the condition of having an illness or disease for which there is no treatment or cure available; the expected outcome is death.

Testosterone is a hormone produced in high amounts in males and that regulates certain characteristics of muscle-building, sexual organs, hair growth, and the deepening of the voice during puberty.

Toxic refers to a poisonous substance.

U

Urinary incontinence is the inability to control the hold of urine in the bladder.

Urologists are physicians who specialize in the treatment of disorders in the urinary tract, as well as problems in the male reproductive organs.

V

Vaccine is a preparation that contains weakened viruses or bacteria and is administered to a person in order to activate immunity to the disease.

Vascular refers to the blood vessels and circulatory system.

Vertigo is a condition characterized by dizziness.

Visceral refers to the structures inside the body.

Virus is a very small infectious organism that requires a living cell to reproduce.

CHAPTER REVIEW QUESTIONS

Match the correct abbreviations and meanings.

1. dispense as written _____   a. AS
2. no known allergies _____   b. DAW
3. bedtime _____   c. OU
4. left ear _____   d. PO
5. as needed _____   e. HS
6. by mouth _____   f. IVP
7. drop _____   g. PCN
8. penicillin _____   h. APAP
9. intravenous push _____   i. NKA
10. as directed _____   j. NPO
11. acetaminophen _____   k. ASA
12. both eyes _____   l. gtt
13. nothing by mouth _____   m. UD
14. after meals _____   n. PC
15. aspirin _____   o. PRN

Resources and References

1. Facts and Comparisons. "Homepage." January 2004. *http://www.factsandcomparisons.com*
2. Food and Drug Administration. "Homepage." January 2004. *http://www.fda.gov*
3. Web M.D. "Homepage." January 2004. *http://www.webmd.com*
4. Colin, P.H. *Dictionary of Medicine.* 2nd Ed. New York, NY: Fitzroy Dearborn Publishers, 1998.
5. *MacMillan Health Encyclopedia.* Revised Ed., Vol. 1–9. USA: Macmillan Library Reference, 1999.
6. Blachford, S.L. and K. Krapp. *Drugs and Controlled Substances: Information for Students.* New York, NY: Thomsom–Gale, 2003.
7. Lambert, Anita. *Advanced Pharmacy Practice for Technicians.* New York, NY: Thomson Learning, 2002.
8. O'Neil, Maryadele, Ed., et al. *Merck Index: An Encyclopedia of Chemicals, Drugs, & Biologicals.* 13th Ed. New York, NY: John Wiley & Sons, 2001.

Routes and Dosage Formulations

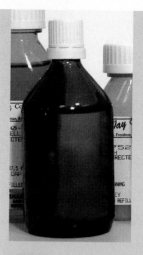

INTRODUCTION

The most common way of taking a medication is orally, or by the mouth. Even though this is the most conventional route of administration, there are many other routes that are used to administer a medication. When people think of medications, their first thought is of a tablet or capsule. These are the most common types of dosage formulations, but may not always achieve the desired results. There are several other dosage formulations that may be more successful in getting the desired effect of the medication. This chapter will introduce the various dosage formulations and routes of administration. We will also look at some common medications in each of these categories. To fully understand a prescription order for administration, we will also look at some common abbreviations used for these routes and dosage formulations.

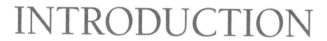

Learning Objectives

After completing this chapter, you should be able to:

- Identify various dosage formulations.
- Identify the advantages and disadvantages of liquid medication dosage formulations.
- Explain the differences between solutions, emulsions, and suspensions.
- Explain the difference between ointments and creams.
- Identify the various routes of administration.
- Give examples of common medications for each route of administration.
- Identify the advantages and disadvantages of each route of administration.
- Identify the parenteral routes of administration.
- Explain the difference between transdermal and topical routes of administration.
- Explain the difference between sublingual and buccal routes of administration.
- Identify the abbreviations for the common routes of administration and dosage formulations.

Dosage Formulations

Medications are available in various dosage formulations. The term dosage form describes how the medication is prepared for administration to the patient. The two primary dosage forms consist of liquid preparations and solid preparations. Common examples of dosage forms include tablets, solutions, suspensions, inhalants, creams, and ointments. A single medication may be available in multiple dosage forms to allow for various disease states, age range, and desired results.

SOLID DOSAGE FORMS

Medications are widely available as solid dosage forms; in fact, most medications are available as a solid form (as well as a liquid form). (See Figure 4-1.) There are different factors to be reviewed when deciding if a solid dosage form is an appropriate choice for the patient. Solid medications may be administered by different routes of administration, such as orally, rectally, vaginally, or topically.

Solid medications have several advantages and disadvantages compared with other forms of medication. Following are some of the common advantages of solid medications:

- Patients are able to self-administer solid medications more easily.
- Solid medications usually have a longer shelf life before expiring.
- Solid medications are easier to package, distribute, ship, and store.
- The dosing is more accurate with solid dosage forms, since the medication is already in a distinctive unit/measure.
- Solid medications usually have little or no taste, compared with the bad taste of liquid medications.
- Solid dosage forms have been created to release the medication over a longer period of time in the patient's body—extended release medications. This allows the patient to take fewer doses, while still getting the same desired effects.

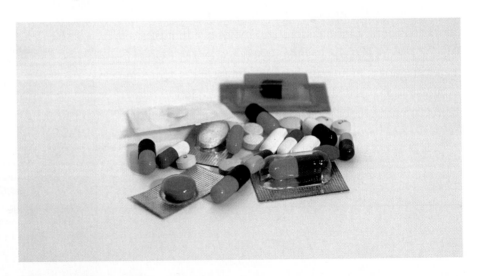

Figure 4-1 Various solid dosage forms

There are also several disadvantages of solid medications:

- Some patients may have difficulty swallowing large tablets or capsules.
- Solid medications are not an appropriate choice for patients who are unconscious or have nasal/mouth breathing tubes for ventilation.
- Solid medications take longer to be absorbed, broken down, and distributed in the body. The stomach has to metabolize the medication before it can take effect.
- Solid medications are not fast enough for immediate action treatments. When immediate action treatments are required, liquids or injectable medications are more appropriate.

Tablets

Tablets are solid medications that are compacted into small, formed shapes. Tablets are usually taken by the mouth for oral administration. Tablets consist of several components. These components work together to ensure that the tablet is properly digested in the body, is easy to swallow, has flavorings or sweeteners for taste, and controls the timed release of the drug to produce the desired effect. All of the ingredients except the active drug are called inactive, or inert, ingredients.

Tablets are classified by the way they are made. The two most common classifications are molded tablets and compressed tablets. Molded tablets are made by using a mold and wet materials. Compressed tablets are formed from die punching compressed, powdered, crystalline, or granular substances into a uniform shape. One characteristic of a compressed tablet is the film, sugar coating, or enteric coating on the outside of the tablet. These outer coverings are commonly used to mask bad-tasting or foul-smelling tablets. They are also used to protect the tablet from the air and humidity. The film coating is used to make the tablet smooth and easier to swallow. Enteric coating is used to protect the tablet from being dissolved in the stomach by the gastric acids. These forms of tablets are used to protect the lining of the gastrointestinal tract and stomach from irritation by the drug. Medications that are to be released over a course of time in the body are made with an enteric coating.

There are five common types of tablets that you need to understand. Each one has unique characteristics and uses.

Chewable tablets are tablets that can be chewed instead of swallowed. Chewable tablet should be chewed, and not swallowed, in order to achieve the desired results. Chewable tablets are most common in pediatric medications, since small children have a difficult time swallowing tablets. Chewable tablets are also known to have sweeteners and flavorings to mask the bad taste and make the medication easier to take. Some adult medications are also chewable, such as antacids and aspirin.

Effervescent tablets are dissolved into a liquid before administration. These tablets contain special ingredients that release the active chemical ingredient by bubbling and fizzing once placed in the liquid. Effervescent tablets have the advantage of being completely dissolved in the liquid before the patient takes the medication. This allows for quicker absorption in the body than a solid tablet.

Sublingual tablets are also quickly absorbed and disintegrated, once placed under the patient's tongue. These tablets are absorbed through the lining of the mouth into the bloodstream.

Buccal tablets are similar to sublingual, except that they are disintegrated in the mouth in the lining of the cheek and then absorbed into the bloodstream. These two types of tablets are useful for medications that are easily destroyed by the stomach acid or poorly absorbed in the bloodstream by the conventional breakdown method.

Vaginal tablets are solid dosage forms that are administered through the vagina. These tablets are dissolved and absorbed through the mucous lining of the vagina. These are useful if immediate treatment and medication is needed in the walls of the vagina.

Capsules

Capsules are solid medication forms in which the drug is contained in an outer coating. Both the active and inactive ingredients are held together by the coating. The most common type of coating is a gelatin shell. The gelatin shells are made of protein from animals. The smooth surface of the gelatin shells allows for easier swallowing.

Gelatin shells are classified into two types: hard and soft. Soft gelatin shells have had ingredients added to the shell to give it a soft, elastic consistency. This allows the capsule to be flexible during administration. The two halves of the soft capsule are sealed together and cannot be broken apart. The shape of soft capsules can vary from round to oblong. They are filled with powdered, pasty, or liquid medications. The soft gelatin capsule is broken apart in the body during absorption to allow the medication to be distributed to the body.

Hard gelatin capsules are characterized by two oblong halves joined together. These capsules are filled with a powdered substance and often intended for oral administration. They are to be swallowed whole. One advantage of a hard gelatin capsule is that it can be broken open and its contents sprinkled over a food substance or into water before administration. This is helpful for patients who are not able to swallow a whole capsule. The ingredients will be dissolved more quickly outside the gelatin shell.

Lozenges

Lozenges are solid dosage forms also known as pastilles or troches. These medications are hard, disk-shaped forms that contain a sugar base. Lozenges are used to deliver a variety of therapeutic remedies to the patient's mouth and throat. Among these remedies are antiseptic, analgesic, anesthetic, antibiotic, decongestant, astringent, and antitussive agents. The lozenge remains in the patient's mouth until it has completely dissolved and released the medication.

Ointments

Ointments are a semisolid dosage form made of solid and liquid medications. Ointments are applied externally to the skin or mucous membranes. They function to deliver a medication to the skin, to lubricate the skin, or to protect the skin. Ointments may or may not contain a medication. They are categorized into the following types: anhydrous, emulsions, oleaginous, or water-soluble. Choosing an ointment depends on the specific characteristics and desired results. Certain medications are more effective in a water-based ointment than in a heavy, greasy base. The different types of ointments are described next.

Oleaginous ointments are emollients used to soothe and cool the skin or mucous membrane. Their primary function is to protect the surface from the air. Their great advantage is being hydrophobic (water repellant) and unable to be washed off. These ointments keep moisture from leaving the skin and therefore are commonly used as lubricants. They can remain on the skin for a long period of time. One disadvantage of oleaginous ointments is their greasy feel.

Water-soluble ointments are the opposite of oleaginous ointments. They are nongreasy to the touch and easily wash off with water. These types of ointments usually do not contain fats or water. Water-soluble ointment bases can be mixed with a nonaqueous or solid medication.

Anhydrous ointments are emollients similar to oleaginous ointments. The major difference between the two ointments is that the anhydrous ointments absorb water instead of repelling it. Anhydrous ointments contain no water. They function to soften and moisturize the skin, but not to the same degree as ointments with an oleaginous base. As they absorb the water, the anhydrous ointment turns into a water-in-oil emulsion.

Emulsions are emollient bases that are comprised of water and oil. The two types of emulsions are oil-in-water and water-in-oil. The water-in-oil bases are heavy, greasy, emollient, and occlusive. The oil-in-water bases are the opposite: water washable, nongreasy, and non-occlusive. These are discussed in detail later in the chapter.

Creams

Creams are semisolid preparations that may or may not contain medication. They can be oil-in-water bases or water-in-oil bases. They are lighter than ointments and can be applied to the skin more easily. Creams function to soothe, cool, dry, and protect the skin. Creams are usually preferred over ointments since they are easier to apply and wash off of the skin.

LIQUID DOSAGE FORMS

Liquid medications are often administered by the mouth in a fluid form consisting of syrups, solutions, emulsions, and suspensions (Figure 4-2). The medium of the fluid serves as a carrier for the medication and is often referred to as the vehicle or delivery system. The vehicle may consist of water

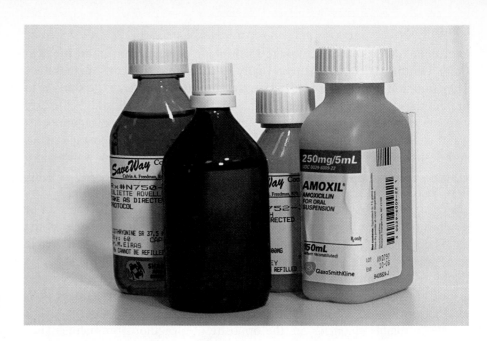

Figure 4-2 Various liquid dosage forms

(aqueous), oil, or alcohol. The medication can be dissolved in the vehicle or remain as a fine solid particle suspended in the fluid. The consistency of the liquid can be as thin as water or thick like syrup.

Liquid medications have several advantages and disadvantages over other forms of medications. The following describes some advantages of the liquid preparations:

- Patients who have difficulty swallowing solid dosage forms such as tablets can better tolerate liquid dosage forms.
- Liquid dosage forms are usually absorbed faster in the body than solid dosage forms. Since the medication is absorbed in the blood-stream as a fluid substance, the body has less to do in order to break it down. Solid dosage forms must be dissolved and broken down in the body before absorption can take place.
- Liquid dosage forms provide more flexibility in achieving the proper dosage and strength of medication. Liquid medications are supplied in bulk preparations and can be measured out more easily than solid medications.

Liquid medications also have several disadvantages over other forms of medications:

- Liquid dosage forms often have a shorter life before expiration than other dosage forms.
- Liquid dosage forms may have a bad taste, as the medication is swallowed or dissolved in the mouth. This may make it especially difficult for children to stay compliant if they don't like the taste of the medication. Sweeteners and flavorings are often used to make liquid medications tolerable for the patient. Solid medications such as tablets and capsules are coated to diminish contact with the taste receptors before they are swallowed.

- Liquid dosage forms may be more difficult to administer for some patients. They can be hard to pour if very thick, and they are often spilled by patients who are physically restrained to some degree.
- Liquid medications usually have special storage requirements that need to be maintained in order for the medication to work properly. Refrigeration is the most common type of storage restriction, and it can be difficult for frequent travelers or school-aged children to comply with.

Solutions are a dosage form in which the medication is completely dissolved and evenly distributed in a homogenous mixture. The molecules of the solid, liquid, or gas medications are equally distributed among the molecules of the liquid vehicle. Solutions are usually absorbed more quickly since the medication is completely dissolved in the liquid mixture. This allows for a more timely effect of the medication. This may be the greatest advantage of solution dosage forms. There are several subcategories of solutions, based on characteristics of the vehicle in which the medication is dissolved. The following will describe these categories in more detail:

Aqueous solutions are liquid mixtures that use purified water as the vehicle. They are available for administration orally, topically, or by injection into the bloodstream. Aqueous solutions are available as douches, irrigating solutions, enemas, gargles, washes, or sprays.

Douches are directed into a body cavity or against a part of the body to clean and disinfect. These can be used to remove debris from the eyes, nose, throat, or vagina. Irrigating solutions are used to cleanse part of the body such as the eye, urinary bladder, or open wounds.

Irrigating solutions are also used to cleanse parts of the body such as the eyes, urinary bladder, abraded skin, or open wounds. These types of solutions contain antibiotics and antimicrobial medications to rid the site of infection. Irrigating solutions are often used over a larger part of the body and in surgical procedures to clear blood and debris.

Enemas are aqueous solutions administered rectally to empty the bowel or treat infections and diseases of the lower gastrointestinal tract. Enemas are usually used to relieve constipation and to cleanse the bowel before a surgical procedure.

Gargles and *washes* are used to cleanse and treat diseases of the mouth or throat. Gargles are held in the patient's mouth to treat throat conditions, such as a sore throat, and then are immediately rinsed. Washes are used more often for cosmetic and disinfecting purposes in the mouth. Similar to gargles, washes are used in the mouth and not swallowed.

Viscous aqueous solutions also use purified water as the liquid vehicle. These liquid preparations are thick, sticky, sweet solutions that may be either liquid or semisolid preparations. These types of solutions include syrups, jellies, and mucilages and are described as follows:

Syrups are concentrated mixtures, with water and sugar used as the dissolving agent. Syrups are distinguished from other solutions by the high concentration of sugar contained in the mixture. There may be medication or flavorings mixed into the syrup. The flavorings or sweeteners are used to flavor the agent and have no medicinal value. These nonmedicated syrups may be used as a vehicle for unpleasant-tasting medications. The biggest advantage of syrup is its ability to cover up the bad taste of a medication. Since the syrup is so thick, only a small portion of the medication comes in contact with the taste receptors in the mouth. Syrups are also characterized by their thick consistency, which has a soothing effect on irritated or infected tissues of the mouth and throat. The most common use of syrups is pediatric and adult cough and cold syrups.

Jellies are semisolid preparations that contain water. These agents are often used as lubricants for surgical gloves, vaginal contraceptive agents, and rectal thermometers. Jellies can be used as lubricants to aide in the insertion and removal of diagnostic probes into orifices or to reduce friction during an ultrasound procedure.

Mucilages are much thicker, viscous, adhesive liquids that contain water and the thick components of vegetable matter. Mucilages are useful to prevent insoluble, solid medication particles from settling at the bottom of the liquid.

Nonaqueous solutions use dissolving agents other than water, although the vehicle may be combined with water. Commonly used vehicles in nonaqueous solvents include alcohol, glycerin, and propylene glycol. The solutions that use only alcohol as the dissolving agent are called alcoholic solutions.

Hydro-alcoholic solutions are nonaqueous solutions. They differ from aqueous solutions in that they contain alcohol in addition to water to act as the vehicle or dissolving agent. Two common examples of hydroalcoholic solutions are elixirs and spirits.

Elixirs are liquid preparations that contain flavored water and alcohol mixtures intended for oral administration. They are clear, sweet solutions that may or may not contain medication. The amount of alcohol component in the mixture will vary, depending on the other ingredients' ability to dissolve easily in pure water. Many drugs dissolve more easily in a water and alcohol mixture than in water alone. The range of alcohol contents in one solution may vary from 2 percent to 30 percent. The greatest advantage of an elixir—the alcohol—may also be its greatest disadvantage. Many patients are not able to consume alcohol, and it may have undesired side effects or interactions with other medications currently being taken. Patients, especially pediatric and elderly, should pay attention to the ingredient contents in elixirs. These populations can be extra sensitive to even the smallest alcohol content. Medicated elixirs are often given to patients who have a difficult time swallowing tablets or capsules.

Two commonly prescribed examples of medicated elixirs are phenobarbital and digoxin elixirs. Elixirs can also be used as sweeteners or flavoring agents. An aromatic elixir is an unmedicated elixir used as a vehicle for other medications. This type of elixir is used to mask the unpleasant taste of the medication. Spirits can have a mixture of alcohol and water, used for easily evaporated substances. Alcohol has a greater concentration and is able to dissolve these substances easier.

Alcoholic solutions contain only alcohol as the dissolving agent. These types of solutions have no water. There may be different types of alcohol used when preparing the solution. The two most common types are ethyl and ethanol alcohols.

Collodions are alcoholic solutions that contain pyroxylin (which is found in cotton fibers) dissolved in either ethanol or ethyl. This liquid preparation is applied to the skin. The alcohol evaporates, leaving only a thin film covering of the pyroxylin. An added advantage of a collodion is the addition of medication. These preparations are used to treat and dissolve corns or warts. A more common example of a collodion is the Band-Aid® liquid bandage, which applies a medication and a thin covering to prevent infection.

Spirits are liquid solutions that may be either alcoholic or hydroalcoholic. Spirits contain volatile, or easily evaporated, substances. Alcohol dissolves these volatile substances more easily than water, allowing a greater concentration of these materials. Spirits may be administered internally or inhaled. Spirits are also known for their flavoring ability, such as peppermint spirits. The most familiar oral spirits are the alcoholic beverages brandy and whiskey. Other spirits may be inhaled through the nose. These are known as aromatic ammonia spirits or smelling salts. If spirits contain water in addition to alcohol, they are identified as hydroalcoholic solutions.

Glycerite solutions are nonaqueous solutions that contain a medication dissolved in glycerin. Glycerin is a sweet, oily fluid that is made from fat and oils. Glycerin is considered a flexible vehicle. It can be used alone or in any combination with water or alcohol. Glycerin is often used as a solvent for medications that do not easily dissolve in water or alcohol alone. Usually, a medication is dissolved in the glycerin, which is then further mixed into a water or alcohol vehicle. Glycerite solutions are often viscous and have the thick consistency of a jelly. Glycerite solutions are rarely used today.

Miscellanous Solutions

Inhalants and *liniments* are commonly used liquid preparations for over-the-counter and prescription medications. Inhalants are medications that contain a fine powder or solution of drugs delivered through a mist into the mouth or nose. The medication immediately enters the respiratory tract for absorption. The most common inhalant medications are inhalers used to treat asthma. Allergy nasal sprays may also be delivered as an inhalant through the nose. Liniments are medications that are applied to the skin with friction and rubbing. Liniments can be solutions, suspensions, or emulsions. Liniments are used to relieve minor cuts, scrapes, burns, aches, and pains. Most liniments contain a medication that produces a mild irritation or reddening of the skin when applied. This irritation then produces a counter-irritation, or mild inflammation, of the skin. This counter-irritation relieves the inflammation of a deeper structure such as tissues or muscles. Ben-Gay® is the most commonly used over-the-counter liniment today.

Emulsions are liquid mixtures of two products that normally do not mix together. One liquid is broken down into smaller elements and even distributed throughout the other liquid. The liquid that was broken down into small elements is called the internal phase, while the other liquid is the external phase. The external phase may also be referred to as the continuous phase since it remains as a liquid substance. Emulsions are named for the emulsifying agent that is used with the two phases. The emulsifying agent is added to the liquid mixture to prevent the internal phase from fusing together and separating from the external phase. If the emulsifying agent is not used, the two liquids will eventually separate and create two distinct layers. This is commonly seen in a bottle of oil and vinegar salad dressing. Before you shake the bottle, you can see the individual layers of oil and vinegar that have separated upon settling. Once shaken, the two layers are mixed together again. This is an example of what happens when an emulsifying agent is not added to the liquid mixture. The two most common forms of emulsions, along with their individual advantages and disadvantages, are discussed next.

Water-in-oil emulsions are liquid mixtures of water droplets distributed throughout the oil substance. These mixtures are commonly used on unbroken skin wounds. Water-in-oil emulsions are spread out more evenly than oil-in-water emulsions, since the skin's natural oils mix well with the external oil phase in the emulsion. The oils also soften the skin better by adding moisture and remaining in the skin when washed with water. These emulsions are often avoided because they easily stain clothing and have a greasy texture.

Oil-in-water emulsions are the opposite of water-in-oil emulsions. These liquid mixtures contain small oil globules dispersed throughout water. These mixtures are commonly used as oral medications. The undesirably oily medications are broken into small particles and dispersed in a sweetened, flavored aqueous vehicle. These small particles are swallowed without contacting the taste buds. The small size of the particles increases absorption in the stomach and bloodstream. Oil-in-water emulsions are lighter and nongreasy. For these reasons, they are the first choice when being applied to a hairy part of the body. The two common types of oil-in-water emulsions are mineral oil and castor oil.

Comparison of Water-in-Oil and Oil-in-Water Emulsions

Each type of emulsion has several advantages and disadvantages. Let's compare the oil-in-water and water-in-oil emulsions.

Several factors are present when choosing the proper emulsion to be used. For irritated skin, the medication is better tolerated if applied to the skin as small particles in the internal phase. The external phase keeps these particles from direct contact with the irritation. The rule of thumb is as follows:

- Medications that dissolve more easily in water are applied as water-in-oil emulsions.
- Medications that dissolve more easily in oil are applied as oil-in-water emulsions.

Suspensions are similar to, but different from, solutions. The particles in solutions are completely dissolved, whereas those in suspensions are not. Suspensions are liquid mixtures with very fine solid particles mixed with a gas, liquid, or solid preparation. Most suspensions are solid particles dispersed in a liquid. A solid medication form may not be appropriate for a particular patient. Since the solid particles in the suspension are very small, the breakdown and absorption process is much quicker than that of tablets or capsules. The medication is in the bloodstream much sooner than it would be if a solid medication form had been used. The key difference between a solution and a suspension is that a suspension must be shaken before use in order for it to redistribute the solid particles that may have settled in the liquid mixture. Suspensions are usually intended for oral ingestion in cases where a large amount of medication is needed. Some suspensions are available for administration by other routes, including ophthalmic, parenteral, otic, and rectal. Suspensions for oral use are combined with water, and the other suspensions may use oil as the vehicle, or dissolving agent.

Magmas and *milks* are suspensions of undissolved medications in water. They are very thick, viscous liquids. These suspensions are intended only for oral use and must be shaken thoroughly before use. Milk of Magnesia® is the most common type of a magma suspension.

Lotions are suspensions for external use only. They are made up of a powdered medication in a liquid mixture. Lotions are used to soothe, cool, dry, and protect irritated skin and wounds. Lotions can function as a disinfectant, protectant, moisturizer, and anti-inflammatory. Lotions have an advantage over other external medications in that they can be easily applied over large areas of the skin. They do not leave an oily or greasy feel on the skin after application. The most common over-the-counter example of a lotion is Calamine® lotion.

Gels are suspensions similar to magmas and milks. The solid particles in gels are much smaller than those in magmas and milks. Gels can be used for oral ingestion. Over-the-counter antacids are common examples of gel suspensions.

Extractives

The last forms of liquid medication we will discuss are liquid mixtures called extractives. Extractives are medications derived from plant or animal tissues. These liquid mixtures are made from concentrated active ingredients from the plant or animal. The drug is withdrawn by soaking the dried tissue in a solvent. Then the liquid is evaporated. The only thing remaining is the active, or crude, drug ingredient. Some examples of extractives are tinctures, extract, and fluidextracts. The various types of extractives are distinguished by their active ingredient potency.

Tinctures are extractives made with alcohol or water solutions. The potency of each mixture is adjusted so that each milliliter of tincture contains the exact same potency of 100 mg crude ingredient. Iodine and paregoric tinctures are two common examples of this type of extractive.

Fluidextracts are more potent than tinctures. Each milliliter of fluidextract contains 1000 mg of the crude drug, as compared with 100 mg in the tinctures.

Extracts are very similar to tinctures and fluidextracts, except for the potency. The highest potent extractive is the extract. The potency of the crude drug in extracts is two to six times stronger than in the others. Common examples of extracts are vanilla, peppermint, and almond extracts used for cooking.

MISCELLANEOUS DOSAGE FORMS

Powders are a solid preparation in which fine particles of active and inactive ingredients are ground up. Powders are usually manufactured and packaged in large supplies for bulk compounding. Powders can be applied internally or externally. Internal administration is done after the powder mixture has been dissolved in a liquid. External powders can be applied directly to the skin to be absorbed into the bloodstream. External powders are also referred to as dusting powders. Commonly used internal powders are potassium supplements that must be dissolved in water or juice for administration. Mycostatin® powder is an external powder used to treat fungal infections on the skin. Powders packaged in bulk supply are difficult to measure accurately. This accuracy is achieved at the individual dose level by packaging the powder in a powder paper, a small piece of paper that measures out exactly one dose. BC Powder® comes packaged in powder papers, each one equivalent to one dose.

Granules are made from powders. The powder is wetted and then dried. Once completely dried, the powder is ground into coarse pieces. Granules are similar to powders, except for their particle size. Powders are ground into much smaller particles than granules. Granules are commonly used in pediatric antibiotic suspensions. Distilled water is added to the package of granules, and the suspension is shaken until the solid particles are completely dissolved in the liquid.

Aerosols are a dosage form in which very fine particles are mixed in a suspension. Inhalers dispense aerosols. The particles can be either liquid or solid. The aerosol mixture is packed with gas and pressure. When used properly, the gaseous pressure forces the liquid or solid particles out of the inhaler and into the respiratory system of the patient. Aerosols can be used for internal or external medications. Internal aerosols are contained in inhalers and can be used in the nose or mouth. The most common example of an internal aerosol is the Albuterol inhaler for asthma. The inhaler forces the medication directly into the lungs and respiratory system so it can immediately provide relief. External aerosols are usually applied topically. Common external aerosols are Tinactin® and Bactine® sprays. One advantage of external aerosols is their ability to be used in hard-to-reach or severely irritated areas of the skin. Aerosols do not cause as much irritation to the wound as other topical treatments such as ointments or creams.

Extended-Release Medications

Some medications are made to be released in the body over a period of time instead of all at once. The medications are referred to as extended-release medications. These types of medications can also be called long acting, sustained-release, or controlled-release. Basically, the medication is absorbed in the body, but only a portion of the active ingredient is absorbed into the bloodstream at a time. Extended-release medications are most commonly available in tablets and capsules. There are a few liquid preparations that are made to slowly release over a period of time. Extended-release medications are available for most of the common illnesses, such as hypertension, diabetes, depression, bacterial infections, and pain.

There are several characteristics and advantages of an extended-release medication. The following are a few that should be considered when selecting an extended-release medication:

- The same amount of medication is released into the bloodstream over a slow, consistent period.
- There is added convenience for the patient. He may have to take fewer doses per day to achieve the same or better results than he would have to take of an immediate action medication.
- Patient compliance will increase with fewer doses and pills to take per day.
- Costs will be lower since not as many pills or doses will be needed. Lower prescription costs also help increase patient compliance.
- Adverse reactions and side effects are reduced, since the medication is slowly introduced into the body.

The extended-release medications are made possible by advanced technologies. Capsules can be made to contain very small beads of medication contained inside a gelatin capsule. The stomach immediately dissolves the gelatin capsule, exposing the beads for absorption. The beads of medication are then dissolved and absorbed over a period of time. Many cold and allergy medications are made in this fashion to provide relief for 6–12 hours after taking one dose. Some extended-release medications are made into two layers. One layer is dissolved and absorbed immediately, while the other one is dissolved gradually over time. Another method of extended-release medications is to embed the medication in a plastic or wax matrix. As the medication is released from the matrix, it is dissolved and absorbed in the body. The matrix itself is not dissolved, but excreted from the body as waste. A more advanced technology uses an osmotic pump to deliver the medication over a period of time. The system consists of a membrane surrounding the medication. Through the process of osmosis, medication is diffused out to the body depending on the concentration. Medication is pushed from the membrane to the body with the entrance and exit of water. The most common example of this type of extended-release medication is Procardia XL®.

Routes of Administration

Medications are delivered to a patient by various forms, more commonly known as routes of administration. Route of administration is the method by which a medication is introduced into the body for absorption and distribution. The route of administration can vary from patient to patient, depending

ROUTES

Route of Administration	Organ of Absorption
Intraocular	Eye
Intranasal	Nose
Buccal	Inside the cheek
Sublingual	Under the tongue
Dermal	Through or in the skin
Inhalation	Lungs
Oral	Stomach and intestine
Intravenous	Venous circulatory system
Intradermal	Dermal layer of the skin
Rectal	Rectum
Vaginal	Vagina
Subcutaneous	Subcutaneous layer of the skin
Intramuscular	Muscle

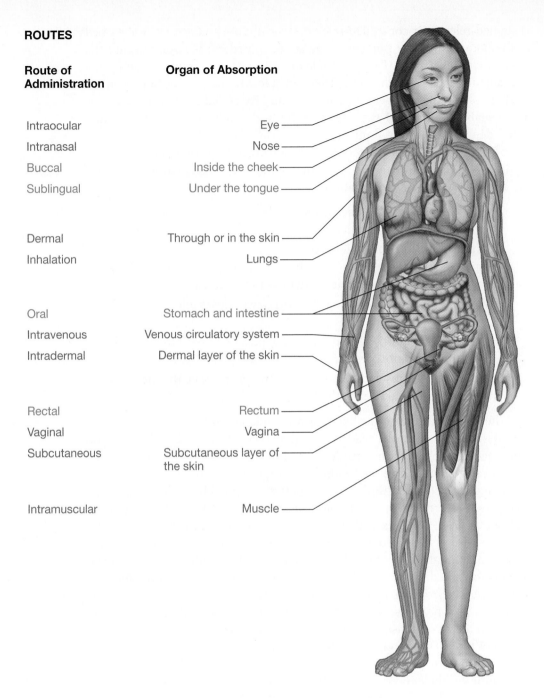

Figure 4-3   Various routes of administration

on the illness. Common examples of routes include oral, topical, parenteral, transdermal, and ophthalmic. (See Figure 4-3.)

The route of administration depends on the desired result of the medication. Several factors are considered when determining the best method to use to deliver a medication to a patient. Consider the following factors for each patient:

- Patient's age—elderly patients may have difficulty swallowing large tablets.
- Patient's physical state—conscience versus unconscious states may determine the best route.
- Patient's medical condition—oral medications may not be used for patients with stomach or gastrointestinal complications.
- Length of time desired to achieve results—injections or IV routes may achieve immediate results better.
- Reduction of side effects—consider possible side effects of different routes.

ORAL

The most common route of administration is oral medications given by mouth. The oral route of administration is abbreviated as PO, derived from the Latin *per os* (by mouth). Capsules, tablets, caplets, liquids, and emulsions are some of the medication dosage formulations that may be taken orally. Most medications are available by an oral route as well as another route. One patient may be treated with an oral tablet or suspension, while another patient may need an injection of the same medication for immediate treatment.

There are several advantages and disadvantages to oral medications. Advantages include the following:

- Oral medications are safe, convenient, and easy to store.
- Oral medications are more readily available in pharmacies. Special injections may have to be special ordered by the physician or pharmacy.
- Oral medications are generally less expensive than other available routes.
- Oral medications are available in immediate-release or extended-release dosage forms.
- Oral medications are easier to administer to yourself, easier for traveling, and generally do not require additional administration supplies.

The disadvantages of oral medications usually lead physicians and patients to choose another route to administer the medication. These disadvantages include the following:

- Oral medications may not be appropriate for children or elderly patients.
- Oral medications may be difficult for patients to swallow if they are unconscious, ventilated, or having digestion problems.
- Unconscious patients cannot swallow anything, so they are generally given medications by injection.

- Oral medications have to be broken down, absorbed, and then distributed to the body. For this reason, oral medications take longer to provide effects and relief.

Oral medications include several distinct types. The most common types are tablets and capsules that are swallowed whole. Oral medications can also be chewed, mixed with a liquid, or completely dissolved before swallowing. Two routes that involve dissolving a medication are buccal and sublingual. Medications given by the buccal route of administration are placed in the mouth, inside the pouch of the cheek. The medication is dissolved and absorbed through the lining of the cheek into the bloodstream. The sublingual route of administration is similar to buccal, except that sublingual medications are placed under the tongue. The medication is dissolved and absorbed through the underlining of the tongue. Medications that are dissolved by these routes provide more immediate relief than swallowing a tablet whole. The most common medication used in the sublingual form is nitroglycerin, given for chest pains.

TRANSDERMAL

Medications delivered across the skin are referred to as transdermal medications. This route of administration is also known as percutaneous. The transdermal route of administration generally uses a patch, which is applied to the skin, where it delivers medication to the bloodstream. In contrast to transdermal medications, topical ointments and creams generally do not deliver medication into the bloodstream; instead, these medications are used for external treatments and protection. There are a few transdermal medications that are made in an ointment or cream semisolid preparation. The most common transdermal ointment is nitroglycerin ointment applied to relieve chest pain.

The patches that are normally used with these medications consist of an adhesive vehicle applied to the skin from which the medication is released into the bloodstream over a period of time. Patches are easy to store, are convenient to use, and remain on the body for a long time. Depending on the medications, patches are made to use for one day or up to a week at a time. Wearing a transdermal patch is considered more convenient than taking a tablet on a daily basis.

There are two types of patches used to deliver transdermal medications. One patch can control the rate of delivery to the skin and bloodstream, while the other patch is designed so the skin controls the rate of delivery. In the patch that controls the delivery, there is a special membrane that is in direct contact with the skin and delivers the medication from a drug reservoir. When the skin is used to control the rate of delivery, the drug is moved from the patch into the blood. The difference in these two routes is the unexpectedly quick delivery of a large amount of medication at once in the second route.

Transdermal patches are becoming more readily available and widely accepted by patients. There are patches available for several different types of medications and uses. Patches are available in the following therapeutic classes: hormone therapy (Climara®, Estraderm®), narcotic analgesics (Duragesic®), birth control (Ortho Evra®), cardiac (nitroglycerin, Catapress®), motion sickness (Transderm Scop®), and medications used to quit smoking (Nicoderm®).

INHALATION

Inhalation is a route of administration by which the medication is inhaled through the mouth and directly absorbed in the lungs. This route of administration is effective for lung conditions when an immediate relief is needed. The most common condition that uses inhalation is asthma. The medication is administered through an inhaler inserted into the mouth. Gases force the medication particles into the mouth and down to the lungs. Other respiratory conditions, such as respiratory infections and congestion, can call for inhalers to help open the lungs and bronchioles if the airways are temporarily constricted. Common examples of medications administered through inhalation include albuterol (Proventil®/Ventolin®), Advair Diskus®, and over-the-counter Primatene Mist®.

NASAL

Medications can be inhaled through the nose also and then absorbed into the bloodstream. Similar to inhalation by mouth, the nasal route of administration provides immediate relief to conditions such as nasal allergies and congestion. The nasal inhaler is held in the nostrils, whereas the liquid medication is sprayed into the nose. There may be additional conditions in which a nasally administered medication is more effective. One example is a narcotic analgesic, Stadol®. When administered nasally, the medication reaches the bloodstream more quickly than through the traditional oral route of administration. Common medications available in nasal route of administration include Flonase®, Rhinocort®, and Stadol®.

PARENTERAL

Besides the oral route of administration, the second most commonly used route of administration is by injection. The definition of parenteral is a route by which the medication does not pass through the gastrointestinal system for absorption and distribution. The top four injection routes are (1) subcutaneous, (2) intravenous, (3) intramuscular, and (4) intradermal. Medications that are delivered by the parenteral routes have several advantages over the oral route of administration. These advantages include quicker absorption and distribution, convenience for patients who cannot take medication by the oral route, and a rate of delivery that can vary from a couple of seconds to several hours. Parenterally administered medications are also very invasive. For this reason, some patients are uneasy with these routes and prefer oral medications. Injections can be very painful for children and the elderly. They also pose an opportunity for bacteria and infection to enter the body.

The common dosage forms of medications given by the parenteral route include suspensions, solutions, and emulsions. Each of the parenteral routes and some common uses and examples of each are discussed next.

SUBCUTANEOUS

The subcutaneous route of administration is one of the most utilized of parenteral routes. The abbreviation for the subcutaneous route is SC. The subcutaneous route is also known as hypodermic injection, since the medication is injected into the tissue immediately under the skin. (See Figure 4-4.) The medication is then absorbed in the bloodstream and distributed to the body where needed. The subcutaneous route delivers the medication at a slower rate than other parenteral routes, such as by the vein or heart muscle. One advantage of the subcutaneous route is the ability for patients to self-administer these types of injections. This route may also be the least invasive parenteral route. Because the medication is not being delivered too far into the body, a smaller needle can be used than is used in other parenteral routes. One disadvantage of the subcutaneous route is the limitation of the volume of the drug that can be injected under the skin. If a large volume is needed, the intravenous route is usually preferred. Many diabetic patients give themselves daily subcutaneous injections of insulin.

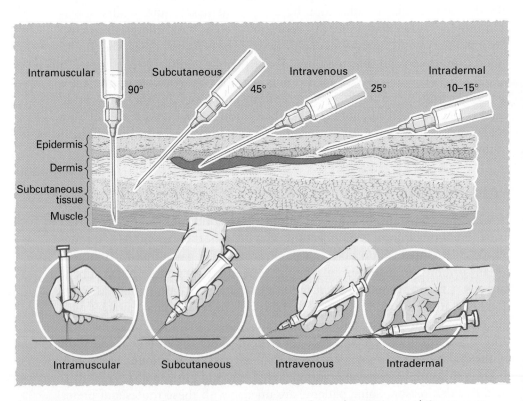

Figure 4-4 Routes of administration—intramuscular, subcutaneous, intravenous, intradermal

INTRAVENOUS

The most common parenteral route of administration is the intravenous route. A medication administered intravenously is injected directly into the vein (Figure 4-4). The medication can be a solution or suspension. The most familiar medical procedure with this route is the I.V. (also the abbreviation for intravenous). Whenever you think of an I.V. infusion, you picture a patient lying in the bed with the I.V. injected into his arm. Intravenous medications can be administered at different rates of delivery. A bolus refers to immediate action after the injection has taken place. A continuous infusion refers to a medication that is released over a period of time following the injection. A common term used for a bolus is I.V. push, which refers to a medication that is pushed into the vein with a syringe. Following an I.V. push, another I.V. can be set up to release over the next few hours. Care must be taken to ascertain the dosages given in I.V. injections. Because the action is immediate, there is little or no time for reversals of any adverse effects. Adverse effects can result from too high of a dose given or not enough of a dose given. Patients who are on a continuous infusion are usually constantly monitored for any abnormal reactions to the medication.

INTRAMUSCULAR

Medications can be injected directly into a large muscle and then absorbed into the body (Figure 4-4). This parenteral route is known as the intramuscular (IM) route of administration. Common dosage forms that can be administered intramuscularly are solutions and suspensions. These are usually injected into large muscle masses such as upper arms, thighs, or buttocks. The medication is absorbed from the muscle and into the bloodstream. These medications are not as quick to work as the intravenous medications. Similar to the I.V. route of administration, the intramuscular rate of delivery can vary from seconds and minutes to a slow infusion over several days. Just like the intravenous route, this route leaves little room for reversal on a medication injected directly into the muscle. Another disadvantage of administering medications intramuscularly is that the injection is usually very painful, causing irritation and pain to the patient.

MISCELLANEOUS PARENTERAL ROUTES

There are several other parenteral routes of administration. Parenteral routes can be applied by injection into almost any area of the body (as opposed to the other routes, which are limited to the skin, arteries, urinary bladder, and abdomen). Let's go over these individual routes and injection sites.

An *implant* is a medical device that slowly releases medication into the body. The implant itself can by inserted as a temporary or permanent device in the body cavity. Implants are often used to treat chronic diseases such as cancer or diabetes. Insulin pumps are implanted in the body to deliver a small amount of insulin as needed. Norplant®, a hormone medication, is

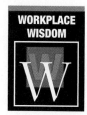

WORKPLACE WISDOM

Determining the gauge and length of a needle is important when preparing medications for injection. Here are some industry guidelines. For I.V. injections—use a 1″ or 1.5″ needle with a 16–20g. For IM injections—again use a 1″ or 1.5″ needle, but with a gauge of 19–22. SC injections are recommended to be given with a $\frac{3}{8}$″ to 1″ needle with a gauge of 24–27.

placed in an implant inserted under the skin in the arm. The implant slowly releases the hormones over a five-year period. At the end of the five years, the implant is removed, and another one is inserted, if desired.

The *intra-arterial* route of administration refers to the method of injecting medications directly into the arteries. This route reduces the risk of adverse reactions and side effects to other parts of the body. There is, however, a greater risk of toxicity if the wrong dosage is administered. Chemotherapy drugs used to treat cancer are commonly administered this way to fight the cancerous agents.

The *intrarticular* route of administration refers to the method of injecting medications directly into the joints. Common injection sites are the elbow and knee. The disease that often calls for the intrarticular route of administration is arthritis. Medications such as Enbrel® and other steroids are used to relieve severe inflammation around the joint.

The *intracardiac* route of administration is used to deliver medications directly to the heart. The medication is injected into the heart muscle. This route is very invasive and only used in cardiac emergencies. The route also poses the risk of rupturing the heart; therefore, it is not highly recommended except as a last resort.

The *intradermal* route injects medications into the top layers of the skin. These injections are not as invasive or as deep as those done by the subcutaneous route. The intradermal route is used to complete skin testing for diseases, such as tuberculosis and allergies to pollens and other microorganisms.

The *intraperitoneal* route is used to inject medications into the abdominal cavity. The abdominal cavity is also referred to as the peritoneal cavity. The common use for this route is to administer antibiotics to treat infections inside the peritoneal cavity.

The *intrapleural* route of administration refers to the injection of medications in the sac surrounding the lungs. These sacs are called pleura. Medications are injected via this route to produce inflammation and scarring of the tissues lining the sacs to prevent excessive fluid build-up from the sacs.

The *intraventricular* route of administration is one of the most invasive parenteral routes. This route is used to inject antibiotics or chemotherapy agents into the brain cavities, or ventricles.

The *intravesicular* route is a less invasive and more common route. When this route is used, a medication is injected directly into the urinary bladder. This route is used to treat urinary bladder infections as well as bladder cancer.

The *intravitreous* route is used to administer medications directly into the eye. Most medications do not reach the eye from the bloodstream, so for severe infections of the eye, this route is preferred to directly inject the antibiotic into the eye. Because this route is invasive, it is usually used only for severe diseases that are significantly reducing a patient's sight.

The *intrathecal* route of administration is used to inject medications into the space surrounding the spinal cord. Again, this is a very invasive procedure. It is used to treat infections or cancerous cells of the central nervous system.

TOPICALS

Medications that are administered externally to the skin are referred to as topicals. Topical medications are applied to the surface of the skin and absorbed into the mucous membrane. The mucous membrane usually prevents the medication particles from being absorbed into the bloodstream. For this reason, medications administered topically are usually not intended to treat internal conditions. They are used to cool, soothe, dry, cleanse, disinfect, and protect the skin. Dosage forms that are administered topically include ointments, creams, lotions, and emulsions. Since these medications are not entering the bloodstream, they are made of a higher concentration than those that do enter the bloodstream. Topical medications can be used to treat a simple external skin rash or a slightly deeper skin layer infection. Common examples of medications administered topically include hydrocortisone creams, corticosteroid ointments, and topical antibiotic ointments.

RECTAL

Medications that are administered through the rectum use what is referred to as the rectal route of administration. Medications administered by this route can be a solid, liquid, semisolid, or aerosol. Common dosage forms used rectally include suppositories, enemas, and aerosol foams. After rectal administration, the medication is absorbed into the lower gastrointestinal tract, or the bloodstream to treat other conditions. Rectally administered medications are often used for children when an oral medication is not appropriate. Patients may also prefer a rectally administered medication to treat conditions when they cannot tolerate swallowing a medication. For example, rectal suppositories are commonly used to treat severe nausea and vomiting when the patient is not able to keep the solid medication down. Elderly patients who have difficulty swallowing tablets may also prefer rectally administered medications. Some common examples of medications administered rectally include Phenergan® suppositories, Fleet® Enemas, and Proctofoam®.

VAGINAL

Medications that are inserted into the vagina for absorption and distribution use what is referred to as the vaginal route of administration. Types of dosage forms that can be administered vaginally include solutions, suppositories, tablets, and topical creams or ointments. The most common use for these medications is to treat vaginal infections. Some medications can be administered through the vagina to deliver medication to the bloodstream to treat systemic conditions. Common examples of vaginally administered medications are Terazol®, Mycostatin® tablets, AVC® vaginal suppositories, and Massengill® douches.

OPHTHALMIC

Medications that are administered through the eye use the ophthalmic route. These medications can be a solution, ointment, suspension, or gel. Ophthalmic medications are used to directly treat conditions of the eye such as allergies, infections, conjunctivitis, inflammation, or glaucoma. This direct route has the advantage over an oral medication that has to be absorbed and distributed throughout the entire body because it provides quicker relief than the systemic approach. Medications such as Visine® eye drops relieve itchiness, redness, and swelling conditions of allergies immediately. Ophthalmic medications are also generally very easy to self-administer. They are usually very convenient and easy to store. Common examples of medications delivered through the ophthalmic route include Visine®, Xalatan®, and antibiotic drops.

OTIC

Medications that are administered in the ear are said to use the otic route of administration. These medications are delivered into the ear canal to treat infections, inflammation, and severe wax build-up. Common dosage forms that can be administered through the otic route are solutions and suspensions. These medications are directly absorbed in the ear canal to provide immediate relief.

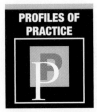

PROFILES OF PRACTICE

The need for a variety of alternative dosage forms is not exclusive to humans. Animals need variety, too! Think of trying to give a cat a capsule by mouth—depending on his mood, it probably is not going to happen. Specialty pharmacies can, however, compound the prescribed medication into a transdermal gel that the owner can simply rub onto the back of the feline's ear. There are also other alternative dosage forms used for animals that we did not list in the chapter. For example, sometimes it is necessary to use a fish or a mouse as the dosage format for patients such as dolphins and snakes.

CONCLUSION

This chapter has reviewed the common dosage forms and routes of administration. Most medications can be delivered through multiple dosage forms and routes. It is important to dispense the proper dosage form of medication; otherwise, a patient may not be able to take the medication as the physician instructed. Diligence regarding the parenteral routes of administration can be crucial to a patient. Some of the parenteral routes can have the same abbreviation, but different meanings. If the wrong route is used, toxicity can result, and there is usually very little that can be done to reverse the injection. It is also very important to administer the correct dose of the medication. Too much or too little can be harmful to the patient.

As a pharmacy technician, you will be working with the pharmacist to prepare and dispense medications to patients. You must understand the meaning of and use for each dosage form and route. Most of the dosage forms imply a certain route to be used. For example, a tablet is commonly administered orally, but it can be administered vaginally as well. Liquid medications can be administered a variety of ways. If the prescription order is not clear as to the dosage form and route, the pharmacist and physician must work together to determine the best method for the patient.

CHAPTER REVIEW QUESTIONS

1. Which of the following is not a type of liquid dosage formulation:
   - **a.** aqueous solution
   - **b.** cream
   - **c.** emulsion
   - **d.** enema

2. Which of the following is an example of a liquid dosage formulation:
   - **a.** tablet
   - **b.** cream
   - **c.** ointment
   - **d.** lotion

3. A parenteral route of administration is one that:
   - **a.** bypasses the gastrointestinal system for absorption.
   - **b.** passes through the gastrointestinal system for absorption.
   - **c.** requires several hours for absorption.
   - **d.** passes through the skin to aid absorption.

4. All of the following are examples of a tablet, except:
   - **a.** buccal
   - **b.** vaginal
   - **c.** lozenge
   - **d.** sublingual

5. The difference between creams and ointments is:
   - **a.** Ointments are a semisolid dosage form that are composed of a solid and liquid medication.
   - **b.** Creams are a semisolid dosage form that may or may not contain a medication.
   - **c.** Creams are usually easier than ointments to apply and wash off the skin.
   - **d.** All of the above are true.

6. Which should not be considered when choosing a route of administration?
   - **a.** patient's age
   - **b.** physical state
   - **c.** medical condition
   - **d.** All of the above should be considered.

7. An extended-release medication is one that:
   - **a.** will not cause drowsiness.
   - **b.** exits the body quickly after absorption.
   - **c.** passes through the digestive system before absorption.
   - **d.** All of the above are true.

8. A subcutaneous injection is:
   - **a.** injected directly into the bloodstream for absorption.
   - **b.** injected into the muscle for absorption.
   - **c.** injected under the skin for absorption.
   - **d.** injected directly into the affected site for absorption.

9. The difference between sublingual and buccal routes of administration is:
   - **a.** The buccal route of administration is where the medication is dissolved and disintegrates in the lining of the cheek.
   - **b.** The sublingual route of administration is where the medication is dissolved and disintegrates in the lining of the cheek.
   - **c.** The sublingual route of medication is one in which the medication is dissolved under the tongue.
   - **d.** Both a and c are correct.

10. Which of the following is not an advantage of a solid medication:

a. has a longer absorption and distribution time in the body

b. easier to package, distribute, ship, and store

c. usually has little or no taste

d. easier to swallow for elderly and disabled patients

Resources and References

1. Ansel, H.C. *Introduction to Pharmaceutical Dosage Forms.* Philadelphia, PA: Lea & Febiger, 1995.

2. The American Medical Association. *Know Your Drugs and Medications.* New York, NY: The Reader's Digest Association, 1991.

3. Facts and Comparisons. "Homepage." January 2004. *http://www.factsandcomparisons.com*

4. Food and Drug Administration. "Homepage." January 2004. *http://www.fda.gov*

5. American Pharmacist Association. *The Pharmacy Technician.* 2nd Ed. Englewood, CO: Morton Publishing, 2004.

6. Hillery, Anya M., Ed., et al. *Drug Delivery and Targeting: For Pharmacists and Pharmaceutical Scientists.* New York, NY: Taylor & Francis, 2001.

7. Lambert, Anita. *Advanced Pharmacy Practice for Technicians.* New York, NY: Thomson Learning, 2002.

8. O'Neil, Maryadele, Ed., et al. *Merck Index: An Encyclopedia of Chemicals, Drugs, & Biologicals.* 13th Ed. New York, NY: John Wiley & Sons, 2001.

Anatomy
and Physiology

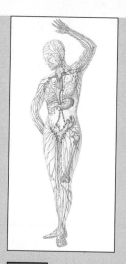

After completing this chapter, you
should be able to:

- Define what constitutes a drug.
- Compare the differences
  between legend and OTC
  medications.
- Describe the principle of
  pharmacology.
- Define and compare the
  processes of absorption,
  distribution, metabolism, and
  elimination.
- Describe the regulatory
  functions of the body.
- Describe the basic human cell
  structure and cell division.
- Explain the basic anatomy and
  physiology of the major
  systems of the body.

INTRODUCTION

Simply put, pharmacology is the study of drugs and their effects on
the human body. As the saying goes, "It takes two to tango." Drug
and body interactions are a two-way street. First there is how the
drug affects the body, known as pharmacodynamics; then there is
how the body affects the drug, known as pharmacokinetics.
Pharmacology is the study of both of these relationships.

Drugs

Drugs, or medications, are substances that diagnose, cure, relieve, treat, or prevent disease. Simply, drugs affect our bodies or our body's processes. In the practice of pharmacy, we deal with two basic types of drugs: prescription and OTC. Pharmacy technicians have to have a working knowledge of both to be effective.

PRESCRIPTION DRUGS

Prescription drugs are those medications that can be addictive, easily abused, or are unsafe unless used under the supervision of a prescriber. The federal government lists these medications—thus the term "legend" drug. Only a licensed prescriber can write prescriptions for these drugs, and these drugs can be dispensed only by a licensed pharmacist.

OTC DRUGS (OVER THE COUNTER)

OTC medications are those that the government feels are safe when the clear and concise directions on the package are followed by the average adult. Many people have the misconception that OTC medications are harmless because they do not require prescriptions. This is a very dangerous misconception. It is important that the patient's profile reflect any OTC drugs he may be taking and that the pharmacist is made aware of that profile, so that proper DUR (drug utilization review) and counseling can take place and be effective. OTC drugs are also subject to the laws prohibiting pharmacy technicians from providing any advice or counseling.

A Drug's Journey through the Body

Proper medication of any patient requires careful monitoring of the absorption, distribution, metabolism, and elimination of drugs. These processes are directly connected to the therapeutic effect the medication will have on the body. Other issues, such as tolerance and abuse (or dependence), are also affected by these processes.

HOW A DRUG ENTERS THE BODY

How a drug enters the body is called the route of administration. This can be through the mouth (oral), lungs (inhalant), eyes (ophthalmically), ears (otically), nose (nasal), skin (transdermal), rectum (rectally), or vaginal (vaginally); or injected through the skin in several ways (injection). It is imperative that the pharmacy technician be familiar with the routes of administration and that he prepare the medications properly.

ABSORPTION

Regardless of how the drug enters the body, it generally cannot work until it enters the bloodstream. This process is referred to as absorption. Since the most common route is oral, the medication must pass through the intestines to be absorbed into the bloodstream. Other routes of administration, such as injections, don't use the intestines and therefore skip the "first pass" stage.

BIOAVAILABILITY

The amount of a drug that eventually becomes available to the body, along with the rate of absorption, is known as bioavailability. Several factors can affect the bioavailability of a drug to the body. These factors include the age, sex, weight, disease state, and genetics of the patient.

DISTRIBUTION

Once the drug is in the bloodstream, how does it get to where it is needed? That process is called distribution. By this stage, the drug is in its molecular stage and can cross cell membranes.

METABOLISM

After the drug has completed its task, it must be prepared for elimination. The liver, kidney, and lungs are the biggest processors; however, other organs can and do help. Metabolism occurs when the body, using enzymes, breaks the drug down into smaller particles called metabolites that are more easily eliminated. While most metabolites are inactive, some metabolites have therapeutic properties after they go through metabolism. Some drugs, called pro-drugs, can be administered in an inactive form and metabolized into an active form.

ELIMINATION

Once the medication has been reduced to metabolites, it needs to be eliminated. Feces and urine are the routes of elimination that come to mind at first, but there are several other ways a body can rid itself of waste or foreign matter. Tears, breath, and sweat are all different ways that a body handles elimination. Without elimination, the medications could build to toxic levels in the body and do significant damage, up to and including death.

Anatomy and Physiology

The basis of anatomy and physiology is the concept of form versus function, as well as the collaborative effort of both. The anatomy is the form, and the physiology is the function. These components work together with the other mechanisms of the body, including body chemistry. A basic knowledge of body chemistry is necessary when attempting to understand the forms and functions of the human body.

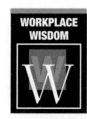

WORKPLACE WISDOM

The term anatomy is derived from the Greek word meaning dissection. It encompasses both the structure of living beings and the study of such structures.

Regulatory Functions of the Body

Homeostasis is the condition in which various factors of the body's internal environment are maintained at relatively stable levels that are suitable to support life. It is regulated by negative feedback systems that consist of receptors, control centers, effectors, and the pathways that connect them. A negative feedback system is a sensing mechanism that is able to identify a change outside particular limits. A control center assesses the change and activates a response to correct or regulate the condition. The control center, also known as the integrator, is often the brain; however, there are many other control centers in the body that regulate various other functions. The stability of the human body relies on the many receptors and the control centers to monitor the conditions necessary to maintain life.

An example of a homeostatic device is a thermostat that regulates the internal temperature of our homes. When it is too cold, we can turn the dial on the thermostat, which signals the furnace to produce more heat. Our bodies have an automatic thermostat that is regulated by our brains. When a person is too hot or too cold, the body's instinctive thermostat is signaled by the mechanisms that maintain normal body temperature. As body temperature increases, the brain detects change and causes increased sweating and dilatation of the blood vessels in the skin. The sweating and increased blood flow cause increased heat loss, enabling the body temperature to return to normal. When the body temperature drops too low, the brain detects the change and causes constriction of the skin and blood vessels, and shivering ensues. The shivering that occurs produces heat, and the decreased blood flow helps retain the heat.

Carbohydrates, Lipids, and Proteins

Every day, we ingest substances that are necessary for our growth and nourishment. Have you ever thought about what the foods you eat consist of? The components in the food you eat can be categorized into three main groups: carbohydrates, lipids, and proteins. Your body requires these staples of life because they give you energy and allow for cellular growth and sustenance. Each category serves a different function in the body.

Carbohydrates, put simply, are sugar molecules. They are sometimes referred to as saccharides. Carbohydrates are used by the body as a quick source of energy. There are three groups of carbohydrates: monosaccharides, disaccharides, and polysaccharides. Monosaccharides contain only one sugar molecule. These are referred to as "simple sugars." Examples of monosaccharides are glucose and fructose. Disaccharides are slightly more complex; these are two linked saccharide molecules. Usually, disaccharides result from a combination of two monosaccharides. Fructose combines with glucose to produce the disaccharide sucrose. The most intricate carbohydrate is the polysaccharide, which is formed from repeated units of monosaccharides that are linked together. The most common polysaccharides are starch and glycogen. Starch is chain of thousands of linked, repeating monosaccharides.

Lipids are another very important building block in the body. A lipid is a substance that is insoluble in water and in some other solvents such as ether. Like carbohydrates, there are three main categories of lipids: triglycerides, phospholipids, and steroids. Lipids are classified into these groups on the basis of their molecular structure. A triglyceride molecule looks different from a phospholipid and a steroid molecule. Triglycerides and phospholipids are metabolic fuels that enable the continual functions of the body systems.

Steroids are interesting because they serve versatile purposes in the body. Examples of steroids are cholesterol, estrogen, and testosterone. Cholesterol is produced by the liver and the cells lining the gastrointestinal tract and is released into the blood. People not only generate cholesterol themselves, but ingest it in the foods they consume (called dietary cholesterol).

Cholesterol is seen as the precursor to the cell membranes, steroid hormones, bile salts, and other specialized molecules. Cholesterol has many important roles in the body; however, it can also cause problems. High concentrations of cholesterol increase the development of arterioscleroses—arterial thickenings that can lead to heart attacks, strokes, and other forms of cardiovascular damage. This is due to high deposits of low-density lipoproteins on the arterial walls in the heart. This type of cholesterol is known as LDL and is deemed the "bad" cholesterol.

The "good" cholesterol is the high-density lipoproteins, or HDL. Doctors use what is called the plasma ratio to determine the likelihood of developing arterioscleroses. This is tested through blood work. Adjusted diet and increased exercise are the first steps that are recommended if a patient's cholesterol needs to be lowered. If these do not prove to have any effect on the plasma ratio, a physician may choose to start the patient on drug therapy to lower the risk of strokes and heart attacks.

Estrogen and testosterone, even though they are considered steroids, are also classified as hormones. These particular steroids are essential in the differentiation between the body chemistries of men and women. Estrogen is the female sex hormone, and testosterone is the male sex hormone. Both are extremely crucial in human reproduction as well as in the development of physical characteristics that distinguish the male and female genders.

Proteins are large molecules composed of one or more amino acids that are joined by peptide bonds. They account for approximately 50 percent of the organic material in the body and about 17 percent of body weight. Proteins are involved in almost all physiological processes that occur in the body. The subunits that constitute proteins are called amino acids. The presence of amino acids makes protein molecules distinct.

The Basic Human Cell

The smallest functional building block of life is the cell. (See Figure 5-1.) Cells perform many essential metabolic functions in the body and are able to communicate with each other through genetic directives, such as deoxyribonucleic acid (otherwise known as DNA) and ribonucleic acid (RNA). These are called nucleic acids since they are located in the nucleus of the cell.

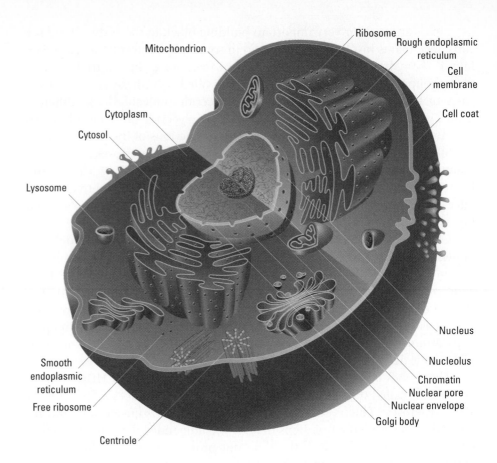

Figure 5-1   A human cell

CELLULAR TRANSPORT

There are two distinct methods of movement of substances into, out of, and between cells. These methods are known as active and passive transport. Without the means of transport, cellular function would not thrive. In both types of transport systems, something known as a concentration gradient is present. This is very important because, depending on the flow of material—either with the gradient or against the gradient—the gradient direction denotes the kind of transport that is taking place. Both active and passive transport can be broken down even further into various subdivisions. We will first begin with the functionality of, and reasons for, passive transport and then progress to the active transport system.

PASSIVE TRANSPORT

The basis of the passive transport process is grounded in the conservation of energy. No energy is expended in this process. This means that the flow of substances is downward. When substances flow down a concentration gradient, there is no consumption of energy. This is a small part of the homeostatic system that was mentioned in the beginning of the chapter. The body uses its own built-in systems to regulate the consumption of energy. Examples of passive transport are bulk flow of materials, diffusion, and osmosis.

Bulk flow is a collective movement of substances in the same direction in response to a force such as pressure. Hence, the movement of blood through the body is an example of bulk flow. No energy is used in the transportation of blood, due to the constant pressure maintained by the body.

Diffusion is the total movement of substances from an area of higher concentration to an area of lower concentration. Again, since this process is passive, the transportation is flowing down, or with, the concentration gradient. Diffusion is the result of the constant and random behavior of the molecules in the body. The molecules consume the energy, resulting in the overall movement of other materials in the body.

Osmosis is a precise type of diffusion. It refers to the movement of water molecules across a selectively permeable membrane. This type of diffusion creates a pressure buildup in the body when it is transferred in. This pressure is called hydrostatic, or osmotic, pressure. Osmosis often occurs in the kidneys, which regulate the osmotic pressure of the body.

ACTIVE TRANSPORT

As we know, the active transport process uses energy to move substances into, out of, and between cells. Active transport is the movement of materials against a concentration gradient and therefore requires the expenditure of energy. There are two mechanisms through which active transport is achieved: (1) transport proteins and (2) vesicles or other bodies contained by the cell.

The transport proteins located in the cytoplasm of the cell transfer material into and out of the cell, as well as within the structure of the cell. Such materials are amino acids, ions, and monosaccharides.

The second method of active transport of the cell deals with the movement of large particles, otherwise known as macromolecules, across the plasma membrane. There are two types of vesicular transportation: endocytosis and exocytosis.

In the process of endocytosis, the plasma membrane plays an important role in the transportation process. The membrane surrounds the substance it is to consume by merging around it and engulfing it. The substance, now surrounded by a vesicle, enters the cytoplasm of the cell. There are three types of endocytosis: (1) phagocytosis, (2) receptor-mediated endocytosis, and (3) pinocytosis.

Phagocytosis occurs when there are undissolved materials inside the cell. The plasma membrane engulfs the materials as in normal endocytosis, but in this case it forms what is known as a phagocytic vesicle. This vesicle, in turn, breaks down the solid material so that it can be used by the cell. Phagocytosis is also called "cellular eating."

Tissues

Cells are arranged into four basic types of tissues that form and assemble organs. The only way to determine which cells make up certain tissues is to study them on a microscopic level. The study of tissues on a microscopic level is called histology. This section explores the four types of tissue and the general characteristics of each. This is a necessary foundation to the later sections dealing with organs and organ systems.

Tissues are groups of similar cells performing a common function. The four categories of tissues are (1) muscle tissue, (2) nervous tissue, (3) epithelial tissue, and (4) connective tissue. These four groups of tissue have subcategories that classify them even further.

There are three types of muscle tissue: skeletal muscle, cardiac muscle, and smooth muscle. Even though all are muscle tissue, each has its own distinct characteristics.

Skeletal muscle tissue is composed of long cylindrical cells that, when viewed under a microscope, appear striated with bands that are perpendicular to the length of the cell. Multinucleated cells are located along the tissue perimeter near the plasma membrane. The skeletal muscles are attached to bones and allow for body movement. These types of muscles are under the conscious control of the brain and are therefore known as voluntary muscles.

Cardiac muscles are also striated like the skeletal muscles; however, they are not multinucleated. They contain a centrally located nucleus with muscle fibers branching off frequently. The cardiac muscles are located only in the heart.

Smooth muscles, like cardiac muscles, contain a centrally located nucleus. They are not striated like the cardiac and skeletal muscles. They are made of elongated cells that taper at the ends. Smooth muscles are found in organs and are known as involuntary muscles. This means that they function automatically without any conscious thought. For example, organs of the digestive and respiratory systems are made up of smooth muscle.

Nervous tissue is made up of two kinds of nerve cells, neurons and neuroglia, also referred to as glial cells. The neuron is the basic structural unit of the nervous system. Each neuron is composed of the cell body (which contains the nucleus), along with other various organelles, dendrites, and an axon. Dendrites are typically short, wiry extensions of the cell body and receive stimuli. The axon is a longer extension of the cell body and sends the stimuli. Neuroglias provide the support system for the neurons. They insulate and anchor the neurons to the blood vessels.

Epithelial tissue, or the epithelium, has general characteristics that make it unique and distinct from the other tissue types. The epithelium consists of tightly packed, flat cells that have scarce internal cellular material. The tissue is avascular, which means that there are no blood vessels present. The exchange of waste and nutrients is carried out through the neighboring connective tissues by diffusion. The surface of the epithelium is exposed to the outside of the body or to the internal body cavity. Thus, the skin that shields and protects the body is made up of epithelial tissue. The cells in the epithelial tissue divide often to replace damaged tissue. This occurs when the outside surface of the body is damaged (as when a person gets a scrape or cut).

There are four types of cells that can compose epithelial tissue: (1) stratified squamous, (2) stratified cuboidal, (3) stratified columnar, and (4) transitional epithelium. All four cellular types are distinct.

Stratified squamous are located beneath the top layer of the skin tissue. They have centrally located nuclei and are closely packed and oblong in shape. They serve as the first layer of protection if the outer layer of the skin is penetrated.

The next layer of epithelial tissue is made up of the stratified cuboidal cells. These cells are usually found in two layers and have centrally located, spherical nuclei. Their function is in secretion and absorption.

The stratified columnar cells are many-sided and several layers thick. They are elongated in shape, similar to columns, and have oval shaped nuclei. They function in secretion and protection.

The transitional epithelial cells vary in shape, depending on the degree of stretching of the skin. They are most often round and large. They also have centrally located nuclei and function only in processes that involve distention or inflation (such as bladder functions).

Connective tissues serve three primary purposes in the body: nerve supply, blood supply, and structure. They do not function alone, but rather work with other tissues and systems in the body. For example, connective tissue is responsible for anchoring other tissues in the body, such as the epithelial tissues, as well as for facilitating the functions of other tissues—for instance, nervous tissues.

In regard to blood supply, the connective tissues of the body are intertwined with a vast vascular system containing blood vessels. This sets the connective tissues apart from the other tissues mentioned. It is the job of the connective tissues to distribute blood flow to other tissues. The connective tissue is doing this job when it works in conjunction with the epithelial and nervous tissues, since those tissues are avascular.

Connective tissue also provides form and structure. The tissues contain scattered cells submerged in cellular material known as the matrix. The matrix consists of fiber and ground substances that define the matrix of the tissue, therefore defining the type of connective tissue.

There are 12 types of connective tissue, of which we will touch only on four: cartilage, bone, blood, and lymph.

Cartilage is a dense type of connective tissue, where the matrix is firm and almost semisolid, allowing for structure and flexibility. Cartilage is primarily made of collagen, which provides its elastic capabilities as a connective tissue. Cartilage is found throughout the body in such places as the ears, nose, and knees. These structures of the body are flexible, yet maintain a firmness. It is the cartilage that is attached to the bones that allows the free movement.

Bone tissue is also a form of connective tissue. Bone tissue is rigid and made up of calcified, ground substances that make the tissue inflexible. Bone tissue provides the unyielding structure of the skeletal system and is the site for attachment of muscle tissue.

Blood and lymph work together as connective tissues. Most people do not think of blood as a "tissue" because it is not a solid substance; however, blood has the characteristics of tissue. Blood and lymph contain cells, just like the previously mentioned tissues. They appear to be liquids, but they do contain cells and fibers.

Blood is composed of three types of cells; leukocytes, erythrocytes, and thrombocytes. The erythrocytes are considered the "red blood cells" and are responsible for the blood's rich red color. The fibers contained in the blood are soluble proteins that form during the clotting process. This makes the matrix of the blood a liquid blood plasma.

Blood functions in several ways as connective tissue. It transports nutrients and oxygen to all of the body's cells and organs. By doing this, it connects the cells, other tissues, and organs, therefore serving its purpose as a connective tissue.

Lymph tissue is similar to the blood in the sense that it also contains soluble protein fibers that form during clotting and has a matrix of liquid blood plasma. Lymph also contains cells known as leukocytes. It does not contain any erythrocytes or thrombocytes, so the lymph appears clear to white in color. The lymph travels through the body, picks up toxins and bacteria, and carries them to structures called lymph nodes that filter, produce antibodies for, and destroy the bacteria.

Integumentary System

The skin that covers the body is considered an organ and a body system. The technical name for the skin is the integumentary system (Figure 5-2). The skin consists of two layers, the epidermis and the underlying dermis. It is regarded as an organ because it contains two types of tissues: connective and epithelial. These tissues were mentioned in the previous section; here, the ways the tissues of the body come together and form organs will be presented, beginning with the form and function of the skin as an organ and protective barrier.

The skin performs a variety of functions, such as protection, sensation, thermoregulation, vitamin metabolism, and excretion.

The skin serves as a protective barrier against ultraviolet radiation, physical damage, and biological invasions (such as by bacteria). It also is a primary sense organ that detects touch, pain, and heat from the nerve endings. The skin uses a system of thermoregulation that works with the homeostatic system. Thermoregulation is supported through the regulation of blood flow to the skin and through sweating, which is also used for the excretion of small waste products such as urea and ammonia. The metabolism of vitamin D occurs in the skin. When natural sunlight is exposed to the skin, vitamin D, which is essential for the growth and development of bone tissue, is produced.

As you can see, the skin plays a vital role in the overall health of the human body. Most people take their skin for granted by abusing it and neglecting it. Proper hygiene is necessary because the skin can become clogged just as a drain can. Any waste that is excreted, if left on the skin, can clog the tiny pores, causing dermatological problems. Poor hygiene also allows bacteria to remain on the skin. This is especially troublesome when bacteria remain on the hands. Bacteria can be transferred to the inside of the body through the eyes, ears, nose, and mouth if they come in contact with the hands.

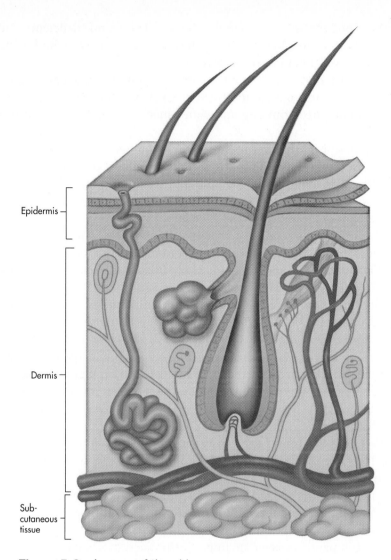

Epidermis

Dermis

Sub-
cutaneous
tissue

Figure 5-2 Layers of the skin

Acne vulgaris, or acne, as it is usually referred to, is an infection of the skin that results from overactive sweat glands. Acne usually occurs in pubescent adolescents, but adults can get it, too. It can cause discomfort and embarrassment for those suffering from the condition. The skin reacts by fighting the infection, by means of the white blood cells. This is why, when a pimple or blemish appears, it sometimes develops a white "head." The pimples that are white in color are considered bacterial infections that begin beneath the first layer of skin. The darker "blackheads" are surface blemishes that are the result of clogged pores. Dermatologists recommend that people do not squeeze blemishes on the face or body, because scarring can occur.

Though sunlight is good for the skin, it can also be very dangerous. Too much sunlight can cause premature wrinkling and, eventually, skin cancers. On the other hand, not enough sunlight can cause a vitamin D deficiency. Vitamin D regulates the growth, hardening, and repair of bones by controlling the absorption of calcium and phosphorus from the small intestine. Osteomalacia, or rickets, is one of the worst possible effects of a vitamin D deficiency. Rickets causes pain in the ribs, lower spine, pelvis, and legs. People who live in low sunlight environments most often develop this disorder.

To prevent a deficiency, supplemental vitamin D can either be taken in capsule form or consumed in foods such as fish and fortified dairy products. However, premature wrinkling and skin cancer are extremely hard to treat and eradicate.

The epidermis is the first layer of skin, contains five sublayers, and suffers the most damage and abuse. It serves as the first barrier of protection. The epidermis is made up of the stratified squamous epithelium that contains four cell types in the five sublayers: (1) keratinocytes, (2) melanocytes, (3) Langerhans cells, and (4) Merkel cells.

The keratinocytes produce a protein called keratin. This protein hardens and waterproofs the skin. The mature keratinocytes are located at the skin's surface. They are dead and almost entirely filled with keratin. Calluses and dry, rough, cracked skin are composed of keratin.

Melanocytes produce a pigment called melanin that protects the skin from ultraviolet radiation. Melanin from the melanocytes is transferred to the keratin. Melanin, one of the components responsible for skin coloration, is activated by sunlight. This is why light-skinned people get a tan and their skin darkens when in the sun. Darker skinned people also get a darker pigmentation in their skin when exposed to sunlight for extended periods, but it is not as noticeable.

Langerhans cells are a type of cell called macrophages or "cell eaters." These cells work along with the white blood cells during an immune response.

Merkel cells are found deep in the epidermis near the boundary of the dermis. They are disclike in shape and, along with the nerve endings, perform sensory functions.

The dermis is the second layer of skin, composed of various connective tissues. There are two sublayers of the dermis: (1) the papillary layer and (2) the reticular layer.

In the thin papillary layer are fingerlike projections called dermal papillae that project into the epidermis above. The dermal layer in the feet and hands contain papillae; the ones in the fingers create the epidermal ridges that define an individual's fingerprints. The reticular layer lies beneath the papillary layer and is much thicker. This portion makes up the majority of the dermis.

There is one more section of the integumentary system, called the hypodermis. The hypodermis is located between the epidermis and dermis, as well as in the underlying tissues and organs. Most of a person's fat is stored here. Its function is to fasten the skin to the supporting surface, absorb shock and impact to the skin, and provide thermal insulation.

The Cardiovascular System

In this section, we will explore the three main functions of the cardiovascular system, as well as detail the flow of blood through the chambers of the heart. The main organ in this system, the heart, will be discussed in detail, along with the three types of blood vessels and how blood flows through the body. This section will close with the mechanisms that aid in the regulation of blood pressure.

Knowing and understanding the functions of the cardiovascular system is key in understanding the general physiology of the human body. This life-sustaining system pumps the blood throughout the body via an extensive structure of veins, arteries, and capillaries. Without the cardiovascular system, a person cannot live.

The cardiovascular system consists of the heart, blood vessels, and blood. The three main functions are to transport, protect, and to regulate. (See Figure 5-3.)

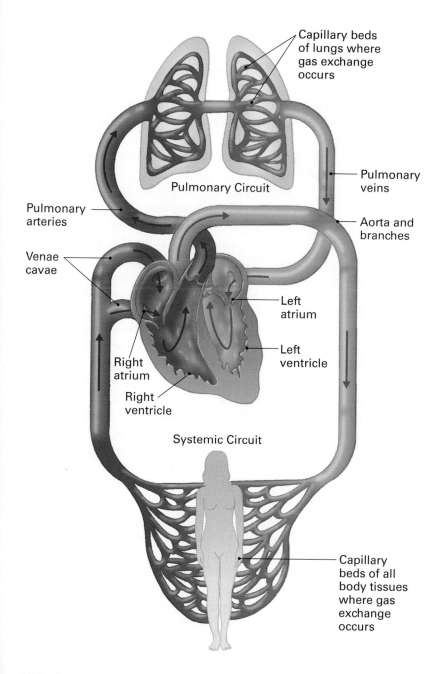

Figure 5-3   The circulatory system

The system transports oxygen, nutrients, and hormones to cells throughout the body. The transport function also serves to remove metabolic wastes. Examples of these wastes are carbon dioxide and nitrogenous waste.

Protection of the body is carried out through the antibodies, white blood cells, and proteins that continuously circulate in the blood. These cells, proteins, and antibodies defend the body against foreign microbes and various toxins. There are also built-in clotting mechanisms that prevent blood loss after the body sustains injury.

Not only does the cardiovascular system transport and protect, but it regulates as well. The system helps regulate the body temperature (via the homeostatic responses, as previously discussed), as well as the pH and water content of the cells.

The blood was classified earlier as a connective tissue. While this is true, it serves many more functions as a part of the cardiovascular system. Blood is composed of cells and cell fragments (called formed elements) and water that contains dissolved molecules, which is called blood plasma.

There are many types of cells in the blood: leukocytes, neutrophils, eosinophils, basophils, lymphocytes, thrombocytes, and monocytes. Each of these cells works together and performs specific functions.

As you know, the erythrocytes are the red blood cells that contain hemoglobin. More than 99 percent of the blood is composed of erythrocytes. These cells function in the transport of oxygen and carbon dioxide.

The leukocytes are a type of white blood cell. They play an important role in the body's immune system, along with functioning in wound healing. Neutrophils are similar to leukocytes in that they function in immunity. Neutrophils, the most common type of white blood cell in vertebrates, are responsible for protecting the body against infection. Staining cells is necessary in some instances because they can be very hard to view under a microscope. Since white blood cells have little to no color, this is necessary. Neutrophilis are stainable with neutral dyes.

Agranulocytosis is a serious blood disorder that occurs when bacteria-destroying white cells (neutrophils) stop circulating in the blood. Symptoms include fever, sore throat, and muscle weakness. This life-threatening condition results from bone-marrow damage caused by certain drugs or by radiation. It is treated with antibiotics and, sometimes, transfusion of white blood cells.

Eosinophils are also another type of white blood cell that is stained with the dye eosin. It is thought that these cells play a part in allergic reactions and immune responses to parasitic diseases.

Basophils are synthesized forms of the common leukocytes. They can be generally classified as white blood cells, or what are called mast cells. In the body, basophils function primarily during allergic reactions. In response to certain stimuli, these cells release a chemical called histamine, which immediately effects a dilation of the blood vessels. This dilation is accompanied by a lowering of blood pressure and an increased permeability of the vessel walls, so that fluids escape into the surrounding tissues. This reaction, the histamine response, may result in a general depletion of vascular fluids, causing a condition known as histamine poisoning or histamine shock. Allergic reactions, in which histamine is released, resulting in the swelling of body tissue, show similarities to histamine poisoning; the two conditions may be associated, and they are treated similarly. The release of histamine is partly responsible for difficult breathing during an asthma attack.

A lymphocyte is a variety of white blood cell consisting of T cells and B cells, both critical to the action of the immune system. T cells directly attack disease-causing bacteria, viruses, and toxins, and regulate the other parts of the immune system. B cells produce antibodies, which neutralize invaders or mark them for destruction by other agents of the immune system. These will be discussed in detail in the section concerning the immune system.

Thrombocytes, or platelets, are the smallest cellular component of blood. They circulate, inactivated, until they meet a damaged blood vessel. At this point, the platelets form a clump, adhering to each other and to the blood vessel wall. They secrete chemicals that alter a blood-borne protein, fibrinogen, so that it forms a mesh of fibers at the damage site. A clot forms when platelets and red and white blood cells become trapped in the fibers. Blood clotting begins within seconds after injury. The same process can produce unwelcome clots in undamaged blood vessels. This may lead to life-threatening occurrences such as strokes.

Monocytes, like many of the previously described cells, are white blood cells that function in the immune response. They attack foreign substances and help identify viruses, harmful toxins, and bacteria.

Blood plasma is composed essentially of water. This watery solution contains small amounts of minerals, salts, sugar (glucose), fats, amino acids, hormones, enzymes, dissolved gases, wastes (similar to urea), and several proteins. One protein is fibrinogen, the substance chiefly responsible for blood clotting. Other important proteins transport crucial chemical elements, such as iron and copper, through the bloodstream, helping to maintain the fluid balance of the body. Plasma proteins known as gamma globulins are antibodies that help protect the body against invasion by bacteria or viruses.

When blood flows past individual cells at the level of the smallest of blood vessels, or capillaries, plasma passes through the capillary walls. The fluid then becomes known as lymph, which is rich in white blood cells. Lymph is much like plasma, except that it contains no proteins, because they are too large to pass through the capillary walls. The lymph delivers the nutrients transported in plasma and collects wastes from the cells. Lymph then rejoins the plasma in the circulatory system so that the wastes can be carried to the organs that excrete them from the body.

Plasma can be separated from blood and used in the treatment of many conditions. It has a longer shelf life than whole blood and, if frozen or dehydrated, can be stored for years. In an emergency, plasma may be more useful than blood because it can be given to anyone regardless of a person's blood type.

Transfusions of plasma may be given to treat shock. Shock occurs when the vital organs are deprived of oxygen-carrying blood. Plasma transfusions restore blood pressure after loss of bodily fluids. Gamma globulin may be extracted from plasma and given to people who have been exposed to such diseases as measles, hepatitis, or mumps.

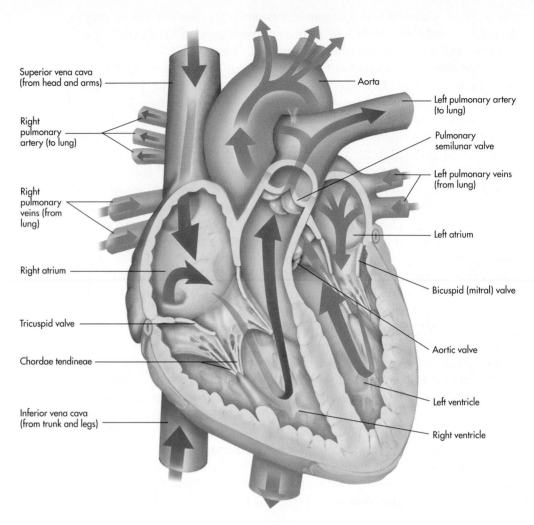

Superior vena cava (from head and arms)

Right pulmonary artery (to lung)

Right pulmonary veins (from lung)

Right atrium

Tricuspid valve

Chordae tendineae

Inferior vena cava (from trunk and legs)

Aorta

Left pulmonary artery (to lung)

Pulmonary semilunar valve

Left pulmonary veins (from lung)

Left atrium

Bicuspid (mitral) valve

Aortic valve

Left ventricle

Right ventricle

Figure 5-4   The heart—the primary organ in the cardiovascular system

Thus far, it is apparent that the elements of the cardiovascular system work together to maintain normal body functions. Although all of the components have their own unique forms and functions, they work together to sustain life. The primary objective when studying anatomy and physiology is to note the forms and functions of elements in the body and understand how they work together as a "team."

The primary organ in the cardiovascular system is the heart (Figure 5-4), is a hollow, cone-shaped muscle located between the lungs and behind the sternum (breastbone). Two-thirds of the heart is located to the left of the midline of the body, and one-third is to the right.

The heart has three layers. The smooth, inside lining of the heart is called the endocardium. The middle layer of heart muscle is called the myocardium. It is surrounded by a fluid-filled sac called the pericardium.

The heart is divided into four chambers: the right atrium (RA), the right ventricle (RV), the left atrium (LA), and the left ventricle (LV). Each chamber has a one-way valve at its exit that prevents blood from flowing backwards into the chamber. When each chamber contracts, the valve at its exit opens. When it has finished contracting, the valve closes so that blood does not flow backwards.

The tricuspid valve is located at the exit of the right atrium. The pulmonary valve is located at the exit of the right ventricle. The mitral valve is located at the exit of the left atrium, and the aortic valve is located at the exit of the left ventricle.

When the heart muscle contracts or beats (identified as the systole), it pumps blood out of the heart. The heart contracts in two stages. In the first stage, the right and left atria contract at the same time, pumping blood to the right and left ventricles. Then the ventricles contract together to thrust blood out of the heart. The heart muscle then relaxes (called the diastole) before the next heartbeat. This allows blood to fill up the heart again.

The right and left sides of the heart have separate functions. The right side of the heart collects oxygen-poor blood from the body and pumps it to the lungs, where it picks up oxygen and releases carbon dioxide. The left side of the heart then collects oxygen-rich blood from the lungs and pumps it to the body so that the cells throughout the body have the oxygen they need to function properly.

All blood enters the right side of the heart through two veins, the superior vena cava (SVC) and the inferior vena cava (IVC). The SVC collects blood from the upper half of the body; the IVC collects blood from the lower half. Blood leaves the SVC and the IVC and enters the right atrium (RA).

When the RA contracts, the blood goes through the tricuspid valve and into the right ventricle (RV). When the RV contracts, blood is pumped through the pulmonary valve, into the pulmonary artery (PA), and into the lungs, where it picks up oxygen.

The blood flows through the heart in this way because blood returning from the body is relatively poor in oxygen. It needs to be full of oxygen before being returned to the body. So the right side of the heart pumps blood to the lungs first to pick up oxygen before going to the left side of the heart where it is returned to the body full of oxygen.

Blood now returns to the heart from the lungs by way of the pulmonary veins and goes into the left atrium (LA). When the LA contracts, blood travels through the mitral valve and into the left ventricle (LV). The LV is a very important chamber that pumps blood through the aortic valve and into the aorta.

The aorta is the main artery of the body. It receives all the blood that the heart has pumped out and distributes it to the rest of the body. The LV has a thicker muscle than any other heart chamber because it must pump blood to the rest of the body against much higher pressure than exists in the general circulation.

A normal, healthy heart is able to maintain a steady beat and rhythm due to a special electrical system that keeps it going.

There are special groups of cells that have the ability to generate electrical activity on their own. These cells separate charged particles. Then they spontaneously disclose certain charged particles into the cells. This produces electrical impulses in the pacemaker cells, which spread over the heart, causing it to contract. These cells do this more than once per second to produce a normal heartbeat of 72 contractions per minute.

The natural pacemaker of the heart, called the sinoatrial node (SA node), is found in the right atrium. The heart also contains specialized fibers that conduct the electrical impulse from the pacemaker (SA node) to the rest of the heart.

The electrical impulse leaves the SA node and travels to the right and left atria, causing them to contract collectively. This takes .04 second. A natural delay allows the atria to contract and the ventricles to fill with blood. The electrical impulse has traveled to the atrioventricular node (AV node). The impulse goes to the bundle of His, and then it divides into the right and left bundle branches, where it rapidly spreads (using Purkinje fibers) to the muscles of the right and left ventricle. This causes them to contract at the same time.

Any of the electrical tissue in the heart has the ability to be a pacemaker. However, the SA node generates an electric impulse faster than the other tissue, so it is in control. If the SA node should fail, the other parts of the electrical system can take over, usually at a slower rate.

Even though the pacemaker cells create the electrical impulse that causes the heart to beat, other nerves can change the rate at which the pacemaker cells fire and affect how strongly the heart contracts. These nerves are part of the Autonomic Nervous System.

The autonomic nervous system has two parts: the sympathetic nervous system and the parasympathetic nervous system. The sympathetic nerves increase the heart rate and the force of contraction; the parasympathetic nerves do the opposite. These activities produce electrical waves that can be measured. The measurement is typically represented as a graph called an electrocardiogram (EKG). Electrical system abnormalities can range from minor premature beats (skipped beats) that do not require treatment to slow or irregular beats that require an artificial pacemaker.

The Brain and the Central Nervous System

The brain, spinal cord, and peripheral nerves make up a complex, integrated information processing and control system called the central nervous system (Figure 5-5). We will examine the structures of the brain and what each one of them does. With this general overview, you will be able to understand concepts such as motor control, visual processing, auditory processing, sensation, learning, memory, and emotions.

The brain is made of approximately 100 billion nerve cells, called neurons (Figure 5-6), which have the amazing ability to gather and transmit electrochemical signals. A neuron has three basic parts: the cell body, the axon, and dendrites (or nerve endings).

The cell body is the main part and has all of the necessary components of the cell: the nucleus, endoplasmic reticulum and ribosomes, and mitochondria. If the cell body dies, the neuron dies.

The axon is a long, cablelike projection of the cell that carries the electrochemical message along the length of the cell. Depending upon the type of

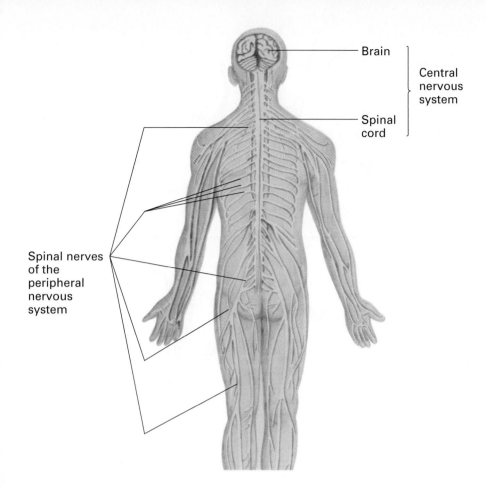

Brain

Central
nervous
system

Spinal
cord

Spinal nerves
of the
peripheral
nervous
system

Figure 5-5 Components
of the nervous system

neuron, axons can be covered with a thin layer of myelin, like an insulated electrical wire. Myelin is made of fat, and it helps to speed transmission of a nerve impulse down a long axon. Myelinated neurons are typically found in the peripheral nerves, which are the sensory and motor neurons, while non-myelinated neurons are found in the brain and spinal cord.

Dendrites (or nerve endings) are small, branchlike projections of the cell that make connections to other cells. Thus, the neuron communicates with other cells or perceives the environment. Dendrites can be located on one or both ends of the cell.

Neurons come in many sizes. For example, a single sensory neuron from your fingertip has an axon that extends the length of your arm, while neurons within the brain may extend only a few millimeters. Neurons have different shapes, depending on what they do. Motor neurons that control muscle contractions have a cell body on one end, a long axon in the middle, and dendrites on the other end; sensory neurons have dendrites on both ends, connected by a long axon, with a cell body in the middle.

Neurons vary not only in size, but also in function. Sensory neurons carry signals from the outer parts of the body (periphery) into the central nervous system. Motor neurons carry signals from the central nervous system to the outer parts (muscles, skin, glands) of the body. Receptors sense

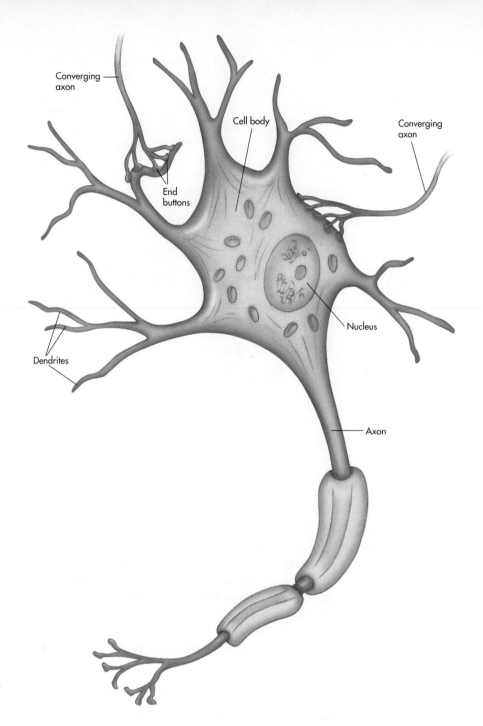

Converging axon

Cell body

Converging axon

End buttons

Nucleus

Dendrites

Axon

Figure 5-6   Structure of a neuron

the environment (chemicals, light, sound, touch) and encode this information into electrochemical messages that are transmitted by sensory neurons. Interneurons connect various neurons within the brain and spinal cord.

The simplest type of neural pathway is a monosynaptic (single connection) reflex pathway. An example of this is the automatic reflex. When the doctor taps the right spot on your knee with a rubber hammer, receptors send a signal into the spinal cord through a sensory neuron. The sensory neuron passes the message to a motor neuron that controls your leg muscles.

Nerve impulses travel down the motor neuron and stimulate the appropriate leg muscle to contract. The response is a muscular jerk that happens quickly and does not involve your brain. Humans have many hard-wired reflexes like this, but as tasks become more complex, the pathway "circuitry" gets more complicated and the brain gets involved.

The simplest creatures have incredibly uncomplicated nervous systems made up of nothing but reflex pathways. For example, flatworms and invertebrates do not have a centralized brain. They have loose associations of neurons arranged in simple reflex pathways. Flatworms have neural nets—individual neurons linked together that form a net around the entire animal.

Most invertebrates, such as the lobster, have simple "brains" that consist of localized collections of neuronal cell bodies called ganglia. Each ganglion controls sensory and motor functions in its segment through reflex pathways, and the ganglia are linked together to form a simple nervous system. As nervous systems evolved, chains of ganglia evolved into more centralized, simple brains.

Regardless of the type of animal, all brains have the same central parts. Understanding the parts of the brain and their primary functions will give you a better understanding of the mechanics of many responses in the body.

The brainstem consists of the medulla, pons, and midbrain. The medulla is an enlarged portion of the upper spinal cord. The midbrain is present only in more advanced animal species. The brainstem controls the reflexes and automatic functions such as heart rate, blood pressure, and limb movements. It also monitors and controls visceral functions like digestion and urination.

The cerebellum integrates information from the vestibular system, which indicates position and movement and uses this information to coordinate limb movements. The hypothalamus and pituitary gland control some visceral functions, body temperature, and behavioral responses such as feeding, drinking, sexual response, aggression, and pleasure.

The cerebrum, also called the cerebral cortex, consists of the cortex, large fiber tracts (corpus callosum), and some deeper structures (basal ganglia, amygdala, hippocampus). It integrates information from all of the sense organs, initiates motor functions, controls emotions, and holds memory and thought processes.

The cerebellum is folded into many lobes and lies above and behind the pons. It receives sensory input from the spinal cord, motor input from the cortex and basal ganglia, and position information from the vestibular system. The cerebellum then incorporates this information and influences outgoing motor pathways from the brain to coordinate movements. To demonstrate this, reach out and touch a point in front of you. Your hand makes one smooth motion. If your cerebellum were damaged, that same motion would be very jerky as your cortex initiated a series of small muscle contractions to hone in on the target point. The cerebellum may also be involved in language (fine muscle contractions of the lips and larynx), as well as other cognitive functions.

The brain is "hard-wired" with connections, much as a building is hard-wired with electrical wiring. In the case of the brain, the connections are made by neurons that connect the sensory inputs and motor outputs with centers in the various lobes of the cortex. There are also connections between these cortical centers and other parts of the brain.

Another section of the brain is called the cerebrum (not to be confused with the cerebellum). The cerebrum has many parts that serve as control centers for language and motor movements. We will now discuss the areas of the cerebrum in order to better explain human language and motions.

The parietal lobe is a portion of the cerebrum that serves specialized functions. It receives and processes all somatosensory input from the body (touch, pain). Fibers from the spinal cord are distributed by the thalamus to various parts of the parietal lobe. The connections form a "map" of the body's surface on the parietal lobe. This map is called a homunculus. The homunculus looks rather strange because the representation of each area is related to the number of sensory neuronal connections and not to the physical size of the area.

The rear of the parietal lobe has a section called Wernicke's area, which is important for understanding the sensory (auditory and visual) information associated with language. Damage to this area of the brain produces what is called "sensory aphasia," in which patients cannot understand language but can still produce sounds.

The frontal lobe is involved in motor skills (including speech) and cognitive functions. The motor center of the brain (precentral gyrus) is located in the rear of the frontal lobe, just in front of the parietal lobe. It receives connections from the somatosensory portion in the parietal lobe and processes and initiates motor functions. Like the homunculus in the parietal lobe, the precentral gyrus has a motor map of the brain.

An area on the left side of the frontal lobe, called Broca's area, processes language by controlling the muscles that make sounds (mouth, lips, and larynx). Damage to this area results in "motor aphasia," a condition in which patients can understand language but cannot produce meaningful or appropriate sounds. Remaining areas of the frontal lobe perform associative processes such as thought, learning, and memory.

The occipital lobe receives and processes visual information directly from the eyes and relays this information to the parietal lobe (Wernicke's area) and motor cortex (frontal lobe). One of the things it must do is interpret the upside-down images of the world that are projected onto the retina by the lens of the eye.

The temporal lobe processes auditory information from the ears and relates it to Wernicke's area of the parietal lobe and the motor cortex of the frontal lobe. The hippocampus is located within the temporal lobe and is important for short-term memory. The amygdala is also located within the temporal lobe and controls social and sexual behavior, as well as other emotions.

The insula influences automatic functions of the brainstem. For example, when you hold your breath, impulses from your insula suppress the medulla's breathing centers. The insula also processes taste information.

The spinal cord can be viewed as a separate entity from the brain or merely as a downward extension of the brainstem. It contains sensory and motor pathways from the body, as well as ascending and descending pathways from the brain. It has reflex pathways that react independently of the brain, such as the automatic reflex.

The Immune System

The concepts and functions of the immune system were briefly addressed in the section on blood. As we learned there, the blood and lymph play important roles in maintaining the overall health of the body. This section will contain some review material as well as new information concerning the body's immune system.

Inside your body, there is an amazing protection mechanism called the immune system. It is designed to defend you against millions of bacteria, microbes, viruses, toxins, and parasites that would love to invade your body. To understand the power of the immune system, all that you have to do is look at what happens to anything once it dies. This shows you something very important about your immune system.

When something dies, its immune system, along with everything else, shuts down. In a matter of hours, the body is invaded by all sorts of bacteria, microbes, and parasites. None of these things is able to get in when your immune system is working, but the moment your immune system stops, the door is wide open. Once you die, it takes only a few weeks for these organisms to completely dismantle your body and carry it away, until all that's left is a skeleton. Obviously, your immune system is doing something amazing to keep all of that dismantling from happening while you are alive.

The immune system is complex, intricate, and interesting; and there are at least two additional good reasons for you to know more about it. First, it is just plain fascinating to understand where things like fevers, hives, and inflammation come from when they happen inside your own body. You also hear a lot about the immune system in the news, as new parts of this complex system are understood and new drugs come on the market. Knowing about the immune system makes these news stories (as well as your profession as a pharmacy technician) understandable.

Each day you inhale thousands of germs (bacteria and viruses) circulating in the air you breathe. Your immune system usually deals with all of them without a problem. Occasionally, a germ gets past the immune system, and you catch a cold, get the flu, or worse. A cold or flu is a visible sign that your immune system failed to stop the germ. The fact that you get over the cold or flu is a visible sign that your immune system was able to eliminate the invader after learning about its presence. If your immune system did nothing, you would never get over a cold or any other ailment.

Along with inhaling germs daily, you eat hundreds of germs; again, most of these die in the saliva or in the acid of the stomach. From time to time, however, one gets through and causes food poisoning. There are normally very visible effects of this violation of the immune system: Vomiting and diarrhea are two of the most common symptoms.

Many human ailments are caused by the immune system working in unexpected or incorrect manners. For example, some people have allergies, which result from the immune system overreacting to certain stimuli that other people do not react to at all. Some people have diabetes, caused by the immune system inappropriately attacking cells in the pancreas and destroying them.

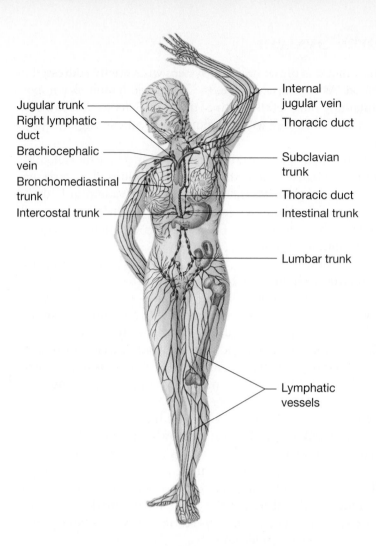

Jugular trunk

Right lymphatic duct

Brachiocephalic vein

Bronchomediastinal trunk

Intercostal trunk

Internal jugular vein

Thoracic duct

Subclavian trunk

Thoracic duct

Intestinal trunk

Lumbar trunk

Lymphatic vessels

Figure 5-7   The principal lymphatic trunks of the body (*Joanna Cameron © Dorling Kindersley*)

Some people have rheumatoid arthritis, an effect of the immune system acting inappropriately in the joints. Many different diseases are actually caused by an immune system error.

There are several components of the immune system that work continually in a healthy individual. Each component has specific tasks to complete as they work together to protect the body. As previously mentioned, sometimes these organ and systems malfunction, causing mild to severe medical problems. The rest of this section looks at each component of the immune system and explores its functions.

The lymph system (Figure 5-7), or lymph, is familiar to people because doctors and mothers often check for "swollen lymph nodes" in the neck. The lymph nodes are just one part of a system that extends throughout your body in much the same way your blood vessels do. The main difference between the blood flowing in the circulatory system and the lymph flowing in the lymph system is that blood is pressurized by the heart, while the lymph system is passive. Fluids ooze into the lymph system and get pushed by normal body and muscle motion to the lymph nodes, very much as water and sewage do in the sewer system in a community.

Lymph is a cloudy liquid that bathes the cells with water and nutrients. Lymph is blood plasma—the liquid and materials that make up blood minus the red and white cells. Blood transfers these materials to the lymph through the capillary walls, and lymph carries it to the cells. As the cells produce proteins and waste products, the lymph absorbs these products and carries them away. Any random bacteria that enter the body also find their way into this intercellular fluid. One job of the lymph system is to drain and filter these fluids to detect and remove the bacteria. Small lymph vessels collect the liquid and move it toward larger vessels so that the fluid finally arrives at the lymph nodes for processing.

Lymph nodes contain filtering tissue and a large number of lymph cells. When fighting certain bacterial infections, the lymph nodes swell with bacteria and the cells fighting the bacteria, to the point where you can actually feel them. Swollen lymph nodes are therefore a good indication that you have an infection of some sort. Once lymph has been filtered through the lymph nodes, it re-enters the bloodstream.

The thymus is located in the chest cavity, between the breastbone and the heart. It is responsible for producing T-cells, and is especially important in newborn babies: Without a thymus, a baby's immune system collapses and the baby will die. The thymus seems to be much less important in adults. For example, you can remove it and an adult will live, because other parts of the immune system can resume the responsibilities of the thymus. However, the thymus is important, especially to T-cell maturation.

The spleen filters the blood by searching out foreign cells and old red blood cells that are in need of replacement. A person missing his spleen gets sick much more often than someone with a spleen. The spleen is not a necessary organ for survival, but an individual with a healthy spleen is usually healthier overall.

Bone marrow plays a very important role in the immune system. Bone marrow produces both red and white new blood cells. The red blood cells are fully formed in the marrow and then are released into the bloodstream. The marrow produces all blood cells from stem cells; the name indicates that they can branch off and become many different types of cells; they are precursors to different cell types. Stem cells change into specific types of white blood cells.

Antibodies, also referred to as immunoglobulins and gamma globulins, are Y-shaped proteins produced by white blood cells. Each antibody responds to a specific antigen (bacteria, virus, or toxin). A special section (at the tips of the two branches of the Y) is sensitive to a specific antigen and binds to it in some way. When an antibody binds to a toxin, it is called an antitoxin. The binding generally disables the chemical action of the toxin. When an antibody binds to the outer coat of a virus particle or the cell wall of a bacterium, it can stop the movement of that invader through cell walls. Large numbers of antibodies can bind to an invader and signal to the complement system that the invader needs to be removed.

The complement system, like antibodies, is a series of proteins. There are millions of different antibodies in your bloodstream, each sensitive to a specific antigen. Only a handful of proteins make up the complement system, which floats freely in the blood. Complements are manufactured in the liver. The complement proteins are activated by, and work with, the antibodies;

hence, they complement them. They cause lysing, or bursting, of cells and signal that a cell needs to be removed.

There are several hormones generated by components of the immune system. These hormones are known generally as lymphokines. Certain hormones in the body, including steroids and corticosteroids (components of adrenaline) suppress the immune system.

Tymosin, thought to be produced by the thymus, is a hormone that encourages lymphocyte production. Interleukins are another type of hormone generated by white blood cells. For example, Interleukin-1 is produced by macrophages after they eat a foreign cell. IL-1 has an interesting side effect; when it reaches the hypothalamus, it produces fever and fatigue. The raised temperature of a fever is known to kill some bacteria.

Sometimes your immune system is not able to activate itself quickly enough to outpace the reproductive rate of a certain bacterium, or the bacterium is producing a toxin so quickly that permanent damage will occur before the immune system can eliminate the invader. In this case, it would be useful to help the immune system by killing the offending bacterium directly.

Antibiotics work on bacterial infections. Antibiotics are chemicals that kill the bacterial cells, but do not affect the cells that make up your body. For example, many antibiotics interrupt the machinery that builds the cell wall inside bacterial cells. Human cells do not contain this machinery, so they are unaffected. Different antibiotics work on different parts of bacterial machinery, so each one is more or less effective on specific types of bacteria. This is because different bacteria have specific structures in the cell wall that are identifiable to certain antibiotics.

One problem with antibiotics is that they lose effectiveness over time. If you take an antibiotic, it will normally kill all of the bacteria it targets over the course of a week or ten days. You will feel better very quickly (in just a day or two) because the antibiotic kills the majority of the targeted bacteria very quickly. However, on occasion, some of the bacterial offspring in the cell wall will remain as mutations that were able to survive the antibiotic. These bacteria will then reproduce, and the whole disease mutates. Eventually, the new strain is infecting everyone exposed to it, and the old antibiotic has no effect. This process has become a reoccurring problem over time, causing significant concern in the medical community.

The Digestive System

The digestive system consists of a series of connected organs whose purpose is to break down, or digest, the food we eat. Food is made up of large, complex molecules, which the digestive system breaks down into smaller, simple molecules that can be absorbed into the bloodstream. The simple molecules travel through the bloodstream to all of the body's cells, where they are used for growth, repair, and energy.

Digestion generally involves two phases: a mechanical phase and a chemical phase. In the mechanical phase, teeth or other structures physically break down large pieces of food into smaller pieces. In the chemical phase, digestive chemicals called enzymes break apart individual molecules of food

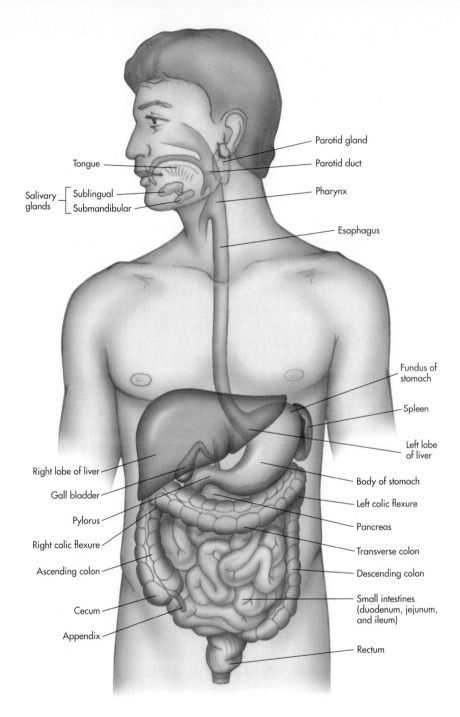

Parotid gland

Parotid duct

Tongue

Salivary glands { Sublingual

Submandibular

Pharynx

Esophagus

Fundus of stomach

Spleen

Left lobe of liver

Right lobe of liver

Gall bladder

Pylorus

Right colic flexure

Ascending colon

Cecum

Appendix

Body of stomach

Left colic flexure

Pancreas

Transverse colon

Descending colon

Small intestines (duodenum, jejunum, and ileum)

Rectum

Figure 5-8 The digestive process

to yield molecules that can be absorbed and distributed throughout the body. These enzymes are secreted by glands in the body.

The process of digestion and the components of the digestive system will now be examined, starting with a brief overview of the system and progressing to specifics. (See Figure 5-8.)

The digestive system consists mainly of a long, continuous tube called the alimentary canal, or digestive tract. This canal has a mouth at one end, through which food is taken in, and an anus at the other end, through which digestive wastes are excreted. Muscles in the walls of the alimentary canal move the food along. Most digestive organs are part of the alimentary canal. However, two accessory digestive organs, the liver and pancreas, are located outside the alimentary canal. These organs contribute to chemical digestion by releasing digestive juices into the canal through tubes called ducts.

Humans digest food entirely through extracellular processes. Food moves in one direction, from mouth to anus, through the series of organs that make up the alimentary canal. Specialization of various parts of the alimentary canal improves the body's ability to break down food and absorb various kinds of nutrients. The mouths of many animals contain teeth designed to break up large portions of food. Behind the mouth, the pharynx and esophagus swallow the food and move it to the stomach. The stomach temporarily stores the food, mixes it with digestive juices, and carries out some digestion.

Digestion is completed in the small intestine. The liver and pancreas pour their digestive juices into the anterior (front) end of this organ. After the anterior intestine absorbs the usable products of digestion, the walls of the posterior (rear) intestine, the large intestine, absorb leftover water. Feces, composed of unabsorbed and indigestible food residues, form in the large intestine, where they are stored until they are excreted through the anus.

If a human adult's digestive tract were stretched out, it would be 6 to 9 meters (20 to 30 feet) long. In humans, digestion begins in the mouth, where both mechanical and chemical digestion occurs. The mouth quickly converts food into a soft, moist mass. The muscular tongue pushes the food against the teeth, which cut, chop, and grind the food. Glands in the cheek linings secrete mucus, which lubricates the food, making it easier to chew and swallow. Three pairs of glands empty saliva into the mouth through ducts, to moisten the food. Saliva contains the enzyme ptyalin, which begins to break down starch.

Once food has been reduced to a soft mass, it is ready to be swallowed. The tongue pushes this mass, called a bolus, to the back of the mouth and into the pharynx. This cavity between the mouth and windpipe serves as a passageway both for food on its way down the alimentary canal and for air passing into the windpipe. The epiglottis, a flap of cartilage, covers the trachea (windpipe) when a person swallows. This action of the epiglottis prevents choking by directing food away from the windpipe and toward the stomach.

The presence of food in the pharynx stimulates swallowing, which squeezes the food into the esophagus. The esophagus, a muscular tube, passes behind the trachea and heart and penetrates the diaphragm before reaching the stomach. Food advances through the alimentary canal by means of rhythmic muscle contractions known as peristalsis. The process begins when circular muscles in the esophagus wall contract and relax one after the other, forcing food downward toward the stomach.

A circular muscle called the esophageal sphincter separates the esophagus and the stomach. As food is swallowed, this muscle relaxes, forming an opening through which the food can pass into the stomach. Then the muscle contracts, closing the opening, to prevent food from moving back into the esophagus. The esophageal sphincter is the first of several such muscles along the alimentary canal. These muscles act as valves to regulate the passage of food and keep it from moving backward.

The stomach, located in the upper abdomen just below the diaphragm, is a saclike structure with strong, muscular walls. The stomach can expand significantly to store all the food from a meal for both mechanical and chemical processing. The stomach contracts about three times per minute, churning the food and mixing it with gastric juice. This fluid, secreted by thousands of gastric glands in the lining of the stomach, consists of water, hydrochloric acid, an enzyme called pepsin, and mucin. Hydrochloric acid creates the acidic environment that pepsin needs to begin breaking down proteins. It also kills microorganisms that may have been ingested in the food. Mucin coats the stomach, protecting it from the effects of the acid and pepsin. About four hours or less after a meal, food processed by the stomach, called chyme, begins passing a little at a time through the pyloric sphincter into the duodenum, the first portion of the small intestine.

Most digestion, as well as absorption of digested food, occurs in the small intestine. This narrow, twisting tube fills most of the lower abdomen. Over a period of three to six hours, peristalsis moves chyme through the duodenum into the next portion of the small intestine, the jejunum, and finally into the ileum, the last section of the small intestine. During this time, the liver secretes bile into the small intestine through the bile duct. Bile breaks large fat molecules into small droplets, which enzymes in the small intestine can handle. Pancreatic juice, secreted by the pancreas, enters the small intestine through the pancreatic duct. Pancreatic juice contains enzymes that break down sugars and starches into simple sugars, fats into fatty acids and glycerol, and proteins into amino acids. Glands in the intestinal walls secrete additional enzymes that break down starches and complex sugars into nutrients that the intestine absorbs. Structures called Brunner's glands secrete mucus to protect the intestinal walls from the acid effects of digestive juices.

The small intestine's capacity for absorption is increased by millions of fingerlike projections called villi, which line the inner walls of the small intestine. Beneath the villi's single layer of cells are capillaries of the bloodstream and the lymphatic system. These capillaries allow nutrients produced by digestion to travel to the cells of the body. Simple sugars and amino acids pass through the capillaries to enter the bloodstream. Fatty acids and glycerol pass through to the lymphatic system.

A watery residue of indigestible food and digestive juices remains unabsorbed. This residue leaves the ileum of the small intestine and moves by peristalsis into the large intestine, where it spends 12 to 24 hours. The large intestine forms an inverted U over the coils of the small intestine. It starts on the lower right-hand side of the body and ends on the lower left-hand side.

The large intestine serves several important functions. It absorbs water and dissolved salts from the residue passed on by the small intestine. In addition, bacteria in the large intestine promote the breakdown of undigested materials and make several vitamins (particularly vitamin K, which the body needs for blood clotting). The large intestine moves its remaining contents toward the rectum, which makes up the final portion of the alimentary canal. The rectum stores the feces until elimination. Then, muscle contractions in the walls of the rectum push the feces toward the anus. When sphincters between the rectum and anus relax, the feces pass out of the body.

The body coordinates the various steps of digestion so that the process proceeds smoothly and cells obtain a steady supply of nutrients and energy. The central nervous system and various glands control activities that regulate the digestive process, such as the secretion of enzymes and fluids. For example, the presence of food in the esophagus, stomach, or intestines triggers peristalsis. Food entering the stomach also stimulates the central nervous system to initiate the release of gastric juice. In addition, as hydrochloric acid passes from the stomach, the small intestine produces secretin, a substance that stimulates the secretion of pancreatic juice.

Certain problems can occur within the digestive system, especially in the intestines, such as diverticular disorders and Crohn's disease. Both affect the intestines; both can become quite painful and inhibit the general quality of life.

The most common symptom of diverticulitis is abdominal pain, and the most common sign is tenderness around the left side of the lower abdomen. If infection is the cause, fever, nausea, vomiting, chills, cramping, and constipation may occur as well. The severity of symptoms depends on the extent of the infection and complications. Diverticulitis can lead to bleeding, infections, perforations or tears, and blockages. These complications always require treatment to prevent them from progressing and causing more serious illness.

Crohn's disease, sometimes called regional enteritis, is a chronic inflammation of the intestines resulting from an extreme reaction of the immune system. The cause is unknown, although there is a genetic tendency to develop this disease and environmental factors are thought to play a part. It may occur at any age, but is most common in young adults, with most people first affected during their teens or twenties.

The symptoms of Crohn's disease include diarrhea, abdominal pain, weight loss, and fever. (Anemia is also caused from bleeding from the intestine, but severe hemorrhaging is rare.) The lining of the intestine becomes inflamed, and ulcers form. Parts of the lining also become swollen, forming a characteristic "cobblestoned" appearance. The muscle wall of the intestine becomes toughened and fibrous, and some areas may become obstructed. Abnormal passages, called fistulae, may form when the inflammation spreads from the intestine through its wall and makes a hole, allowing partly digested or fecal material to pass from the inside of the intestine to another part of the body.

The Urinary System

In this section, the basic aspects of the urinary system as it applies to both men and women will be presented. Men and women have the same basic internal structures of the urinary system.

The urinary system eliminates waste products from the body and maintains the fluid–salt balance. The system consists of paired kidneys with ureters, a urinary bladder, and a urethra. It is sometimes called the excretory system because it excretes waste products from the body. (See Figure 5-9.)

The kidneys are two bean-shaped organs below the ribs in the back of the torso (area between ribs and hips). They are responsible for maintaining the

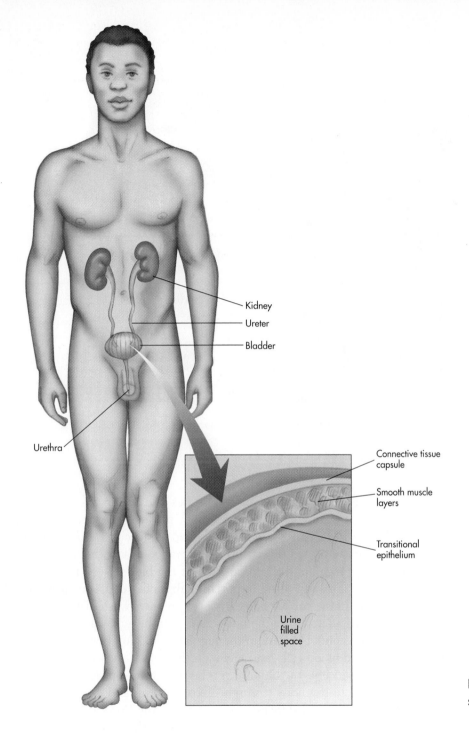

Kidney

Ureter

Bladder

Urethra

Connective tissue capsule

Smooth muscle layers

Transitional epithelium

Urine filled space

Figure 5-9 The urinary system

fluid–salt balance by removing extra water and wastes from the blood and converting them to urine. The kidneys keep a stable balance of salts and other substances in the blood. They also produce hormones that build strong bones and help form red blood cells. Although the kidneys are small organs, they receive a large amount of the blood pumped by the heart. The large blood supply to the kidneys enables them to carry out several tasks.

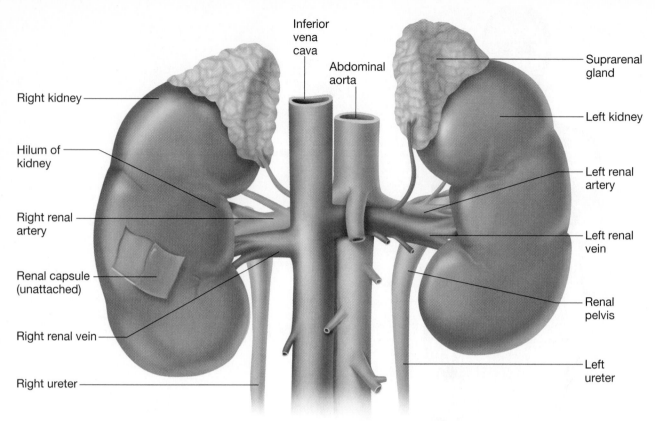

Right kidney

Hilum of
kidney

Right renal
artery

Renal capsule
(unattached)

Right renal vein

Right ureter

Inferior
vena
cava

Abdominal
aorta

Suprarenal
gland

Left kidney

Left renal
artery

Left renal
vein

Renal
pelvis

Left
ureter

Figure 5-10 The kidneys

Urine is carried by narrow, muscular tubes, the ureters, from the kidneys to the bladder, a triangular-shaped reservoir in the lower abdomen. Like a balloon, the bladder's walls stretch and expand to store urine and then flatten when the urine is emptied through the urethra to outside the body.

The kidneys regulate the composition of the blood, keep the concentrations of various ions and other important substances constant, maintain the volume of water in the body at constant levels, remove wastes (urea, ammonia, drugs, toxic substances) from the body, and keep the acid–base concentration of the blood constant. They aid in the regulation of blood pressure, stimulate the making of red blood cells, and maintain the body's calcium levels.

The kidneys receive the blood from the renal artery, process it, return the processed blood to the body through the renal vein, and discard the wastes and other unwanted substances in the urine. Urine flows from the kidneys through the ureters to the bladder. In the bladder, the urine is stored until it is excreted from the body through the urethra. To understand how the kidney does these impressive jobs, you need to take a closer look inside the organ. (See Figure 5-10.)

The cortex and medulla, located inside the kidney, contain many tiny, tubular structures that stretch across both regions perpendicular to the surface of the kidney. In each kidney, there are 1 million of these structures, called nephrons. The nephron is the basic unit of the kidney. (See Figure 5-11.) This

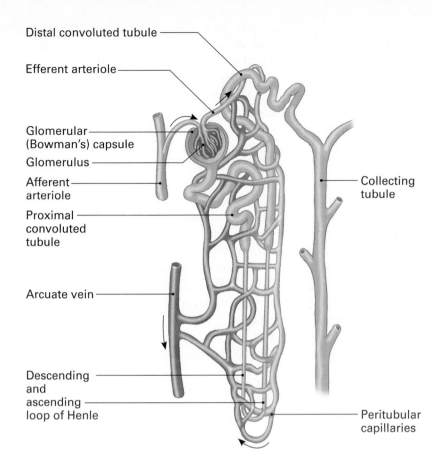

Figure 5-11   The structure of a nephron

Distal convoluted tubule

Efferent arteriole

Glomerular (Bowman's) capsule

Glomerulus

Afferent arteriole

Proximal convoluted tubule

Arcuate vein

Descending and ascending loop of Henle

Collecting tubule

Peritubular capillaries

long, thin tube, closed at one end, has two twisted regions interspaced with a long hairpin loop, ends in a long straight portion and is surrounded by capillaries. The kidney is the only organ of the body in which two capillary beds, in series, connect arteries with veins. This arrangement is important for maintaining a constant blood flow through and around the nephrons despite fluctuations in systemic blood pressure.

Each nephron consists of five major parts. The Bowman's capsule is the closed end at the beginning of the nephron, located in the cortex. The proximal convoluted tubule, or proximal tubule, is the first twisted region after the Bowman's capsule, also in the cortex. The loop of Henle, a long loop positioned after the proximal tubule, extends from the cortex down into the medulla and back. The distal convoluted tubule, or distal tubule, is the second twisted portion of the nephron after the loop of Henle (also in the cortex). Finally, the collecting duct is the long, straight portion located directly after the distal tubule. This is the open end of the nephron, extending from the cortex down through the medulla.

Kidneys regulate blood composition by three major processes: (1) filtration, (2) reabsorption, and (3) secretion. These are vital steps, since the kidneys receive approximately 20 percent of the body's blood supply.

In the nephron, approximately 20 percent of the blood is filtered under pressure through the walls of the glomerular capillaries and Bowman's capsule.

The filtrate is composed of water, ions (sodium, potassium, chloride), glucose, and small proteins. The rate of filtration is approximately 45 gallons (180 liters) each day. The amount of any substance that is filtered is the product of the concentration of that substance in the blood and the rate of filtration. So, the higher the concentration, the greater is the amount filtered (or the greater is the filtration rate), and the more substance is filtered.

This filtration process is much like the making of espresso coffee or cappuccino. In a cappuccino machine, water is forced under pressure through a fine sieve containing ground coffee; the filtrate is the brewed coffee. The arrangement of the glomerular capillaries, in series with the peritubular capillaries, is important to maintain a constant pressure in the glomerular capillaries and thus a constant rate of filtration, despite momentary fluctuations in blood pressure. Once the filtrate has entered the Bowman's capsule, it flows through the nephron into the proximal tubule.

Inside the nephron, small molecules (such as ions, glucose, and amino acids) are reabsorbed from the filtrate. Specialized proteins called transporters are located on the membranes of the various cells of the nephron. These transporters grab the small molecules from the filtrate as they flow by. Each transporter grabs only one or two types of molecules. For example, glucose is reabsorbed by a transporter that also grabs sodium (Na). (See Figure 5-11.)

Transporters are concentrated in different parts of the nephron. For example, most of the Na transporters are located in the proximal tubule, while fewer ones are spread out through other segments. Some transporters require energy, usually in the form of adenosine triphosphate (ATP), while others do not.

Water is reabsorbed passively by osmosis in response to the buildup of reabsorbed Na in spaces between the cells that form the walls of the nephron. Other molecules are reabsorbed passively when they are caught up in the flow of water. The reabsorption of most substances is related to the reabsorption of Na, either directly by sharing a transporter or indirectly by using the flow of the water, which is set up by the reabsorption of Na.

Two major factors affect the reabsorption process: the concentration of small molecules in the filtrate and the rate of flow of the filtrate. The higher the concentration, the more molecules can be reabsorbed. The flow rate affects the time available for the transporters to reabsorb molecules.

The kidneys also have the ability to conserve or to waste water. For example, if you drink a large glass of water, you will find that you will have the inclination to urinate within an hour or so. In contrast, if you do not drink for a while, such as overnight, you will not produce much urine, and when you do, it will usually be very concentrated (darker). Two mechanisms are involved in this process of water balance in the urinary system: the loop of Henle and the antidiuretic hormone (ADH).

The loop of Henle has a descending limb and an ascending limb. As filtrate moves down the loop of Henle, water is reabsorbed, but ions (Na and Cl) are not. The removal of water serves to concentrate the Na and Cl. As the filtrate moves up the other side (ascending limb), Na and Cl are reabsorbed, but water is not. These two transport properties set up a concentration difference in NaCl (sodium chloride) along the length of the loop, with the highest concentration at the bottom and lowest concentration at the top. The loop of Henle can then concentrate NaCl in the medulla. The longer the loop, the larger the concentration gradient will be. This also means that the medulla tissue tends to be saltier than the cortex tissue.

As the filtrate flows through the collecting ducts, which go back down through the medulla, water can be reabsorbed from the filtrate by osmosis. Water moves from an area of low Na concentration (high water concentration) in the collecting ducts to an area of high Na concentration (low water concentration) in the tissue of the medulla. If you remove water from the filtrate at this final stage, you can concentrate the urine.

ADH, secreted by the pituitary gland in the brain, controls the ability of water to pass through the cells in the walls of the collecting ducts. If no ADH is present, then no water can pass through the walls of the ducts. The more ADH present, the more water can pass through.

Specialized nerve cells, called osmoreceptors, in the hypothalamus of the brain sense the Na concentration of the blood. The nerve endings of the osmoreceptors, located in the posterior pituitary gland, secrete ADH if the Na concentration of the blood is high. If the Na concentration of the blood is low, they do not secrete ADH. In reality, there is always at least some very low level of ADH secreted from the osmoreceptors.

A diuretic is a chemical compound that increases the flow of urine and thus eliminates accumulations of water in cells, tissues, blood, and organs. The retention of excess water may occur following injury, as when water accumulates in the knee; in congestive heart failure, when the heart pumps insufficient blood to eliminate a normal volume of fluid; and in a variety of other disabilities, including hypertension (high blood pressure), cirrhosis of the liver, and kidney diseases.

Heart stimulants, such as digitalis, produce a diuretic effect by increasing blood pressure and thus increasing the flow of blood through the kidneys. Certain substances, such as caffeine in coffee and tea, increase urine output by counteracting the tendency of blood proteins to prevent the removal of water from the blood by the kidneys. A class of drugs known as loop diuretics (such as furosemide) is extremely effective when used to increase urine output. All diuretics can have side effects. Diuretics may cause abnormal levels of sodium, potassium, chloride, and other substances.

Problems can occur within the urinary system, especially in the kidneys. One prevalent problem that individuals face is the formation of kidney stones. A kidney stone forms in the kidney when there is an imbalance between certain urinary components—chemicals such as calcium, oxalate, and phosphate. Crystallization is caused by the imbalance; thus, a "stone" is formed.

Caucasians are more prone to develop kidney stones than African Americans. Although stones occur more frequently in men, the number of women who get them has been increasing. Kidney stones occur most typically in people between the ages of 20 and 40. Once a person forms a stone, there is a 50-percent chance that they will develop another stone.

Scientists do not always know what makes kidney stones form. While certain foods may promote stones in susceptible people, researchers do not believe that eating a specific item will cause stones in people who are not vulnerable. Yet, there are factors such as a family or personal history of kidney stones and other urinary infections or diseases. These histories have a definite connection to this problem. Climate and water intake may also play a role in stone formation. Stones can form because of an obstruction to the urinary passage, as in prostate enlargement or stricture disease. Stone formation has also been linked to hyperparathyroidism, an endocrine disorder that results in increased levels of calcium in the urine.

Another condition that can cause kidney stones to form is absorptive hypercalciuria, a surplus of calcium in the urine that occurs when the body absorbs too much calcium from food. The high levels result in calcium oxalate or phosphate crystals forming in the kidneys or urinary tract. Similarly, hyperuricosuria, excess uric acid related to gout or the excessive consumption of meat products, may also trigger kidney stones.

Consumption of calcium pills, certain diuretics, or calcium-based antacids by a person who is at risk to form stones may increase the risk of forming stones by increasing the amount of calcium in the urine. Calcium oxalate stones also may form in people who have chronic inflammation of the bowel or who have had an intestinal bypass operation. This is due to excessive loss of water from the body, as well as absorption of oxalate from the intestine.

The treatment of kidney stones has progressed over the years. Now, laser treatments are available. The patient undergoes a relatively painless procedure to break up the crystallization of the stone into smaller pieces so that it is able to pass through the urethra with relatively less pain. However, surgery is sometimes required for larger stones that cannot be broken up via the laser treatments.

The Respiratory System

The function of the respiratory system is to deliver air to the lungs. The oxygen in air diffuses out of the lungs and into the blood, while the carbon dioxide diffuses in the opposite direction. The carbon dioxide moves out of the blood and into the lungs. This process is called respiration.

Respiration involves several subprocesses. Pulmonary ventilation is the act of inspiration and expiration; put simply, inhaling and exhaling gases, such as those in the air. External respiration is another subprocess involved in the overall respiration of the body. External respiration is the exchange of gases between the lungs and the blood. Gas transport, also vital in respiration, is carried out by the cardiovascular system. Gas transport is the process of distributing oxygen throughout the body, as well as collecting carbon dioxide for removal by the lungs.

Internal respiration, the last component of respiration, is the process of gas exchange between the blood and interstitial fluids (fluids surrounding the cells), on the one hand, and the cells themselves, on the other. It is inside the cell that cellular respiration generates energy (ATP). Internal respiration completes this task by using oxygen and glucose to produce carbon dioxide as a waste product.

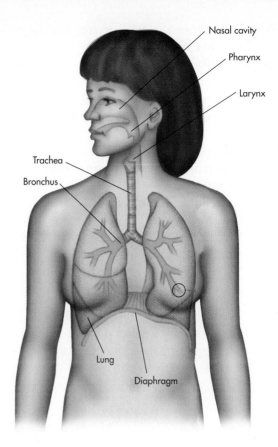

Figure 5-12   The respiratory system

The overall structure of the respiratory system is extensive and complex. The respiratory system works with other body systems to facilitate the life-sustaining processes. (See Figure 5-12.)

The respiratory system will be examined from the intake of oxygen (inhalation), through its gas exchange, transformation to carbon dioxide, and, eventually, the exhalation of the waste product. The primary organs and their structures and functions will also be discussed.

The nose is the site where both the initial inhalation and final exhalation take place. The nose consists of the visible external nose and the internal nasal cavity.

Air enters the nostrils and passes through an area called the vestibule, located just beyond the nostrils. It then moves on through the chambers called meatuses. Meatuses consist of bony walls, called concha, that are formed by facial bones.

From the meatuses, air flows to the right and left chambers of the internal nasal structure. Hair, mucus, blood capillaries, and cilia line the nasal cavity. They perform various functions, such as filtering, moistening, warming, as well as eliminating debris from the passing air.

The pharynx, or throat, has three main regions. The first, the nasopharynx, receives air from the nose. The pharynx, the second region, receives air

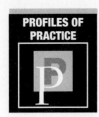

from the nasopharynx, along with food from the oral cavity. The laryngopharynx passes food to the esophagus and air into the larynx.

The next structure in the respiratory system is the larynx, which, as mentioned in the previous section, receives air from the laryngopharynx. The larynx is composed of many parts, as are most structures in the respiratory system. The larynx contains nine pieces of cartilage joined by membranes and ligaments.

The epiglottis, the first piece of cartilage of the larynx, is flexible flap that closes to cover the glottis (the upper region of the larynx) during swallowing to prevent the entrance of food into the airways.

The thyroid cartilage, commonly called the "Adam's apple," protects the anterior portion of the larynx. The pair of arytenoid cartilages located on the posterior portion of the larynx are horizontally attached to the thyroid cartilage in the front by a series of folded mucous membranes.

CONCLUSION

The human body is an amazing machine. In order to better understand drugs and their effects on this miracle of nature, pharmacy technicians must possess at least a rudimentary knowledge of its workings.

CHAPTER REVIEW QUESTIONS

1. The innate system that regulates and maintains normal body function is:
   - **a.** equilibrium
   - **b.** homeostasis
   - **c.** cytokenisis
   - **d.** none of the above

2. Proteins are large molecules that are composed of one or more _____ that are joined by peptide bonds.
   - **a.** monosaccharides
   - **b.** lipids
   - **c.** amino acids
   - **d.** hormones

3. A negative feedback system is a sensing mechanism that is able to sense change _____ particular limits.
   - **a.** outside
   - **b.** inside
   - **c.** beyond
   - **d.** none of the above

4. Carbohydrates are:
   - **a.** fats
   - **b.** meats
   - **c.** salts
   - **d.** sugars

5. Cholesterol is produced by the cells lining the gastrointestinal tract and by the:
   - **a.** liver
   - **b.** heart
   - **c.** kidneys
   - **d.** lungs

6. The most important component of the human cell is the:
   - **a.** plasma membrane
   - **b.** Golgi body
   - **c.** nucleus
   - **d.** mitochondria

7. Groups of similar cells performing a common function are classified as:
   - **a.** cells
   - **b.** tissues
   - **c.** tumors
   - **d.** organisms

8. The basic structural units of the nervous system are called:
   - **a.** muscles
   - **b.** chromatids
   - **c.** axons
   - **d.** neurons

9. The skin that covers the body is considered both a body system and:
   - **a.** an organ
   - **b.** a shield
   - **c.** a sponge
   - **d.** none of the above

10. The smallest cellular components of the blood are:
    - **a.** eosinophils
    - **b.** granules
    - **c.** thrombocytes
    - **d.** neutrophils

Resources and References

1. Reifman, Noah. *Certification Review for Pharmacy Technicians, 6th Ed.* Evergreen, CO: Ark Pharmaceutical Consultants, Inc., 2002.

2. American Pharmacist Association. *Pharmacy Technician Workbook and Certification Review.* Englewood, CO: Morton Publishing, 2001.

3. American Society of Health System Pharmacists. *Manual for Pharmacy Technicians.* Bethesda, MD: ASHP, 1998.

4. American Society of Health System Pharmacists. *Pharmacy Technician Certification Review and Exam.* Bethesda, MD: ASHP, 1998.

5. Ballington, Don. *Pharmacy Practice.* St. Paul, EMC Paradigm, 1999.

6. Ballington, Don. *Pharmacy Practice for Technicians.* St. Paul, EMC Paradigm, 2003.

7. Cowen, D. and W. Helfand. *Pharmacy: An Illustrated History.* New York: Harry N. Abrams, Incorporated, 1990.

8. Lambert, Anita. *Advanced Pharmacy Practice for Technicians.* Clifton Park, NY: Delmar, 2002.

Top 200 Drugs

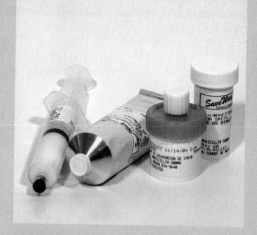

INTRODUCTION

Listed in this chapter are the top 200 most commonly dispensed medications in the United States (Table 6-1). Familiarity with these medications will aid you in assisting both the pharmacist and the patient. Knowing what medications are used for, their brand as well as trade (generic) names, and dosage forms and strengths is important for good pharmacy practice. Every year there are slight changes to this list, but, in general, most of these items will be constant for a number of years. The list is organized by presenting the most commonly dispensed drugs first. Pay close attention to the therapeutic class (usage), as well as the generic names. In addition, you will find a basic overview of the origins, uses, and naming systems of drugs.

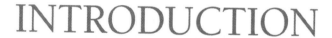

Learning Objectives

After completing this chapter, you should be able to:

- List five origins of drugs.
- Recognize and describe the four types of drug names.
- List the most commonly prescribed medications by both trade and generic names, along with their uses.

TABLE 6-1 Top 200 Drugs

Generic Name	Trade Name	Class and Use	Strength and Form
hydrocodone w/APAP	Anexia, Lortab Lorcet, Vicodin	narcotic analgesic	various, tab
atorvastatin	Lipitor	lipid lowering agent	10, 20, 40 mg tab
levothyroxine	Synthroid	synthetic thyroid hormone	25, 50, 75, 88, 100, 112, 125, 150, 175 200, 300 mg tab
atenolol	Tenormin	adrenoreceptor	25, 50, 100 mg tab
azithromycin	Zithromax	macrolide antibiotic	250, 300, 600, 900, 1200 mg tab, powder for suspension
amoxicillin	Amoxicillin	antibiotic	250, 500, 875 mg tab, 200, 400 mg chewable tab
furosemide	Lasix	diuretic	10, 40, 80 mg tab, 10 mg/ml injection 10 mg/ml oral solution
hydrochlorothiazide	HydroDiuril	diuretic/anti-hypertensive	25, 50, 100 mg tab
amlodipine	Norvasc	calcium channel blocker	2.5, 5, 10 mg tab
lisinopril	Prinivl, Zestril	ACE inhibitor	2.5, 5, 10, 20, 30, 40 mg tab
alprazolam	Xanax	benzodiazepine	0.25, 0.5, 1, 2 mg tab
sertraline	Zoloft	serotonin reuptake inhibitor	25, 50 mg tab
albuterol	Proventil, Ventolin	andrenergic bronchodilator	0.5%/3 ml, 100 mcg inh., 0.83% nebulas, 200 mcg rotocap
metoprolol	Toprol XL	andrenoreceptor blocker	25, 50, 100, 200 mg tab
simvastatin	Zocor	lipid lowering agent	5, 10, 20, 40, 80 mg tab
conjugated estrogen	Premarin	synthetic estrogen hormone	0.3, 0.625, 0.9, 1.25, 2.5 cap
lansoprazole	Prevacid	gastric acid inhibitor	15, 30 mg tab
cetirizine	Zyrtec	H_1-receptor antagonist	5, 10 mg syrup
ibuprofen	Advil, Motrin	NSAID	200, 400, 600, 800 mg tab oral suspension
levothyroxine	Levoxyl	synthetic thyroid hormone	25, 50, 75, 88, 100, 112, 125, 150 175, 200, 300 mcg tabs
propoxyphene NAPAP	Darvocet-N	narcotican analgesic	$\frac{65}{100}, \frac{130}{200}, \frac{195}{300}$ mg tab
triamterene/HCTZ	Maxzide, Dyazide	diuretic/antihypertensive and antikaliuetic agent	$\frac{25}{37.5}$ mg tab
celecoxib	Celebrex	NSAID	50, 100, 200 mg cap
zolpidem	Ambien	non-benzodiazepine and hypnotic	5, 10 mg tab
fexofenadine	Allegra	histamine H_1-receptor antagonist	30, 60, 180 mg tab
cephalexin	Keflex	cephalosporin antibiotic	250, 500 mg tab, oral suspension
esomprazole	Nexium	anti-gastric-acid secretor	20, 40 mg tab
alendronate	Fosamax	inhibits bone resorption	5, 10, 40 mg tab
rofecoxib	Vioxx	NSAID (removed from market 9/30/2004)	12.5, 25, 50 mg tab, oral suspension

TABLE 6-1 Top 200 Drugs (*continued*)

montelukast	Singulair	leukotriene receptor antagonist	10 mg tab, 5 mg chewable tab
norgestimate/ethinyl/ estradiol	Ortho Tri-Cyclen	contraceptive and homone replacement	multiple tab
prednisone	Prelone	adrenal corticosteroid	1, 2.5, 5, 10, 20, 50 mg tab
metoprolol	Lopressor	beta$_1$-adrenoreceptor blocker antihypertensive	25, 50, 100, 200 mg tab
fluoxetine	Prozac	antidepressant	10, 20, 40 mg cap. syrup
venlafaxine	Effexor XR	antidepressant	25, 37.5, 50, 75, 100 mg tab
gabapentin	Neurontin	anticonvulsant and neuropathic pain blocker	100, 300, 400, 600, 800 mg cap, syrup
lorazepam	Ativan	antianxiety agent	0.5, 1, 2 mg tab, 2 mg/ml injection
clonazepam	Klonopin	benzodiazepine	0.5, 1, 2 mg tab
citalopram	Celexa	SSRI	20, 40 mg tab
sildenafil	Viagra	erectile dysfunction	100, 150 mg tab
bupropion HCL	Wellbutrin SR	antidepressant	75, 100 mg tab
paroxetine	Paxil	psychotropic	10, 20, 30, 40 mg tab, oral suspension 12.5, 25 mg CR tab
pravastatin	Pravachol	HMG-CoA reductase inhibitor lipid lowering agent	10, 20, 40 mg tab
clopidogrel	Plavix	ADP adrenosine inhibitor blood clot inhibitor	75 mg tab
amoxicillin	Trimox	antibiotic	oral suspension
potassium chloride	K-Dur	electrolyte (potassium) replenisher	10, 20 mEq tab
pantoprazole	Protonix	gastric acid secretion inhibitor	20, 40 mg tab
salmeterol/fluticasone	Advair Diskus	bronchodilator and corticosteroid	$\frac{100}{500}, \frac{250}{50}, \frac{500}{50}$ mcg diskus
fluticasone	Flonase	corticosteroid	50 UG AQ suspension
metformin	Glucophage	antihyperglycemic	500, 800, 1000 mg tab, 500 mg XR tab
amoxicillin clavulanate	Augmentin	antibacterial	125, 200, 250, 400, 600, 800 mg cap oral solution
amitriptyline	Elavil	antidepressant	10, 25, 50, 75, 100, 150 mg tab
ranitidine HCI	Zantac	histamine$_2$-receptor antagonist	150, 300 mg tab, 150 mg efferdose syrup, injection
acetaminophen/codeine	Tylenol/Codeine	analgesic/antipyretic/ opiate	#2 $= \frac{15}{300}$, 3 $= \frac{30}{300}$, 4 $= \frac{60}{300}$ mg tab, liquid $= \frac{12}{120}$ mg/ml
escitalopram	Lexapro	SSRI	5, 10, 20 mg tab
quinapril	Accupril	ACE inhibitor	5, 10, 20, 40 mg tab

TABLE 6-1 **Top 200 Drugs** (*continued*)

Generic Name	Trade Name	Class and Use	Strength and Form
levofloxacin	Levaquin	broad spectrum antibacterial	250, 500, 750 mg tab
ramipril	Altace	ACE inhibitor	1.25, 2.5, 5 mg tab
valsartan	Diovan	angiotensin antagonist	80, 160 mg tab
amlodipine/benazepril	Lotrel	ACE inhibitor	2.5, 5, 10, 20 mg tab
warfarin	Warfarin	anticoagulant	1, 2, 4, 5, 6, 10 mg tab
omeprazole	Prilosec	gastric acid inhibitor	10, 20 mg cap
cyclobenzaprine	Flexeril	skeletal muscle relaxant	10 mg tab
glipizide	Glucotrol	blood glucose reducer	2.5, 5, 10 mg tab
fluconazole	Diflucan	synthetic antifungal	50, 100, 200 mg tab, oral suspension
verapamil	Calan	calcium channel blocker	120, 180, 240 mg, SR cap
valdecoxib	Bextra	NSAID	100 mg tab
penicillin VK	V-Tids	antibiotic	250, 500 mg tab, 250 mg/ml solution
losartan	Cozar	anangiotensin II receptor antagonist	25, 50 mg tab
pioglitazone	Actos	antidiabetic agent	15, 30, 45 mg tab
trazodone	Desyrel	antidepressant	50, 10, 150, 300 mg tab
glyburide	DiaBeta, Micronase Glynase	blood glucose lowering agent	1.25, 2.5, 5 mg tab
naproxen	Naprosyn	NSAID	375, 500 mg tab
valsartan/HCTZ	Diovan HCT	angiotensin II antagonist	40, 80, 160, 320 mg tab
warfarin	Coumadin	blood thinner	1, 2, 2.5, 4.5, 6, 7.5, 10 mg tab
norelgestromin/ethinyl estradiol	Ortho Evra	contraceptive	tablets, various strengths
rosiglitazone maleate	Avandia	oral antidiabetic	2, 4, 8 mg tab
paroxetine	Paxil CR	psychotropic	12.5, 25 mg tab
risperidone	Riseperdal	psychotropic	0.25, 0.5, 1, 2, 3, 4 mg tab
tamsulosin	Flomax	alpha1A antagonist	0.4 mg tab
rabeprazole	Aciphex	antisecretory	20 mg tab
digoxin	Digitek	cardiac glycoside	125, 250 mcg tab
ciprofloxin	Cipro	fluoroquinolone antibiotic	100, 250, 500, 750 mg tab, oral suspension
mometaxone	Nasonex	nasal anti-inflammatory corticosteroid	100 mg spray
oxycodone/APAP	Oxycodone APAP	non-opiate analgesic and antipyretic	$\frac{5}{500}$ mg tab
metformin	Glucophage XR	antihyperglycemic	500 mg tab
benazepril	Lotensin	ACE inhibitor	5, 10, 20, 40 mg tab

TABLE 6-1 Top 200 Drugs (*continued*)

raloxifene	Evista	estrogen receptor modulator	60 mg tab
olanzapine	Zyprexa	psychotropic	2.5, 5, 7.5, 10, 15, 20 mg tab
diltiazem	Cardizem	calcium channel blocker	30, 60, 90, 120 mg tab
fexofenadine/ pseudoephedrine	Allegra-D	histamine H_1-receptor antagonist	60, 120 mg tab
clonidine	Clonidine	antihypertensive	0.1, 0.2, 0.3 mg tab
digoxin	Lanoxin	cardiac glycoside	125, 250 mcg tab
losartan HCTZ	Hyzar	angiotensin II receptor antagonist and diuretic	25, 50 mg tab
amoxicillin	Amoxil	synthetic antibiotic	250, 500, 875 mg tab, 200, 400 chewable
risedronate	Actonel	antiresorptive agent	5, 30 mg tab
oxycodone	Oxycontin	narcotic analgesic	$\frac{5}{500}$ mg tab
trimeth/sulfameth	Cotrim	sulfanamide	$\frac{80}{400}, \frac{60}{800}$ mg tab
latanoprost	Xalatan	prostaglandin	50 mcg/ml liquid
fenofibrate	Tricor	lipid regulating agent	67, 134, 200 mg tab
glimepride	Amaryl	blood glucose lowering agent	1, 2, 4 mg tab
methylphenidate XR	Concerta	CNS stimulant	18, 36 mg tab
fluticasone propionate	Flovent	nasal anti-inflammatory	nasal spray
glyburide/metformin	Glucovance	antihyperglycemic	$\frac{1.25}{250}, \frac{2.5}{500}, \frac{5}{500}$ mg tab
ipatropium/albuterol	Combivent	anticholinergic/ bronchodilator	$\frac{21}{120}$ mcg inhalant
amphetamine mixed salts	Adderall XR	amphetamine	5, 10, 20, 30 mg tab
omeprazole	Prilosec	antisecretory	10, 20 mg cap
quetiapine	Seroquel	antipsychotic	25, 100, 200 mg cap
drospirenone/ethinyl estradiol	Yasmin 28	oral contraceptive	various
valacyclovir	Valtrex	antiviral	250, 500 mg tab, 1 gm tab
divalproex	Depakote	anti-epileptic, mania, migraine	250, 500 mg cap
conjugated estrogens/ medroxyprogesterone	Prempro	hormone replacement	$\frac{0.625}{2.5}, \frac{0.625}{5}$ mg tab
carisprodol	Soma	muscle relaxant	350 mg tab
isosorbide mononitrate	Imdur	organic nitrate	30, 60, 120 mg tab
levothyroxine	Levothroid	synthetic thyroid hormone	25, 50, 75, 88, 100, 112, 125 mg tab
irbesartan	Avapro	angiotensin II receptor antagonist	75, 150, 300 mg tab
diazepam	Valium	benzodiazepine	2, 5, 10 mg tab oral suspension
tolterodine	Detrol LA	muscarinic receptor antagonist	1, 2 mg tab

TABLE 6-1 Top 200 Drugs (*continued*)

Generic Name	Trade Name	Class and Use	Strength and Form
human insulin NPH	Humulin-N	insulin replacement	unit-measured vial
insulin glargine	Lantus	long-acting insulin replacement	unit-measured vial
carvedilol	Coreg	adrenergic-blocking agent	3.125, 6.25, 12.5, 25 mg tab
enalapril	Vasotec	ACE inhibitor	2.5, 5, 10, 20 mg tab
tramadol/acetaminophen	Ultracet	synthetic analgesic	50 mg tab
promethazine/codeine	Phenergan	antihistaminic sedative	$\frac{6.25}{25}$ mg/5 m syrup, 12.5, 25, 50 mg tab 12.5, 25, 50 mg suppository
oxycodone/APAP	Endocet	antipyretic	$\frac{5}{500}$ mg tab
gemfibrozil	Lopid	lipid regulator	600 mg tab
topiramate	Topamax	antiepileptic	25, 50, 100, 200 mg tab
metaxalone	Skelaxin	muscle relaxant	400 mg tab
clarithromycin	Biaxin XL	macrolide antibiotic	250, 500 mg tab, 125, 250 mg/5 ml suspension
diltiazem	Cartia XT	calcium channel blocker	30, 60, 90, 120 mg tab
monopril	Fosinopril	ACE inhibitor	10, 20, 40 mg tab
ezetimibe	Zetia	lipid lowering agent	10 mg tab
folic acid	Folvite	folic acid replacement	1 mg tab
budesonide	Rhinocort Aqua	anti-inflammatory corticosteroid	$\frac{32}{64}$ mcg
cefdinir	Omnicef	cephalosporin	300 mg cap, 125 mg/5 ml suspension
meclizine	Antivert	antiemenic	12.5, 25, 50 mg tab
triamcinolone acetonide	Nasacort AQ	glucocorticosteroid	55 mcg spray
amoxicillin/clavulanate	Augmentin ES	antibiotic	600 mg tab
nitrofurantoin	Macrobid	bactericidal	25, 50, 100 mg cap
temazepam	Restoril	benzodiazepine hypnotic	7.5, 15, 30 mg cap
doxycycline	Vibramycin	broad spectrum antibiotic	200 mg tab
sumatriptan	Imitrex Oral	antimigraine	25, 50 mg tab
ethinyl estradiol/ norethindrone	Necon	contraceptive	tablets, various strengths
potassium chloride	KCL	potassium replacement	10 mEq tab
potassium chloride ER	Klor-Con M20	potassium replacement	20 mEq tab
allopurinol	Zyloprim	xanthine oxidase inhibitor	100, 300 mg tab, injection
phenytoin	Dilantin	antiepileptic	30, 100 mg cap
trimeth/sulfameth	SMZ-TMP	synthetic antibacterial	$\frac{80}{40}$, $\frac{160}{800}$ tab
norethindrone/ethinyl/ estradiol	Microgestin FE	contraceptive	tablets, various strengths
insulin lispro	Humalog	glucose regulator	100 units/ml, 10 ml vial

TABLE 6-1   Top 200 Drugs (_continued_)

cefprozil	Cefzil	cephalosporin antibiotic	250, 500 mg tab
fentanyl	Duagesic	opiod analgesic	multiple doses/ surface area, patch
mupirocin	Bactroban	antibiotic	20 mg/2% ointment
olopatadine	Patanol	H_1-receptor antagonist	0.1% solution
human insulin $\frac{70}{30}$	Humulin $\frac{70}{30}$	insulin replacement	100 units/ml (U-100)
donepezil	Aricept	enzyme inhibitor	5, 10 mg tab
PEG 3350	Miralax	osmotic agent	powder for reconstitution
levonorgestrel/ethinyl /estradiol	Aviane	contraceptive	multiple, tab
cetirizine/ pseudoephedrine	Zyrtec-D	H_1-receptor antagonist/ adrenergic vasoconstrictor	$\frac{5}{120}$ mg tab
oxybutinin	Ditropan XLO	antispasmodic, anticholinergic	5, 10, 15 mg tab
clarithromycin	Biaxin	macrolide antibiotic	250, 500 mg tab
ciprofloxacin	Cipro	broad spectrum antibiotic	100, 250, 500, 750 mg tab
niacin	Niaspan	niacin replacement	500, 750, 1000 mg tab
atomoxetine	Strattera	norepinephrine reuptake inhibitor	10, 18, 25, 40, 60 mg cap
propranolol	Inderal LA	beta-adrenergic receptor blocker	60, 80, 120 mg cap
pimecrolimus	Elidel	dermatological	1% cream
budesonide	Pulmicort	corticosteroid	200 mcg inhaler
levonorgestrel/ethinyl estradiol	Triphasil-28 Trivora-28	contraceptive	multiple tab
albuterol	Albuterol	$beta_2$-adrenergic bronchodilator	100 mcg/dose aerosol
nifedipine	Nifedipine ER	calcium channel blocker	30, 60, 90 mg tab
methylprednisolone	Medrol	glucocorticoid	2, 4, 8, 16, 24, 32 mg tab
hydrocodone/ chlorpheniramine	Tussionex	narcotic, antitussive, antihistamine	10 mg/5 ml
meloxicam	Mobic	NSAID	7.5 mg tab
timolol	Timoptic	beta-adrenergic blocker	2.5 mg/ml gel
candesartan	Atacand	angiotensin receptor antagonist	4, 8, 16, 32 mg tab
phenytoin	Dilantin	antiepileptic	30, 100 mg cap
brimonidine	Alphagan P	adrenergic agonist	1.5 mg/ml solution
moxifloxicin	Avelox	broad spectrum antibiotic	400 mg tab
clotrimazole/ betamethasone	Lotrisone	antifungal/corticosteroid	$\frac{10.0}{0.64}$ mg/g cream
triamcinolone	Aristocort	glucocorticosteroid	200 mcg aerosol
fluvastatin	Lescol XL	cholesterol lowering agent	20, 40 mg tab

TABLE 6-1   Top 200 Drugs (*continued*)

Generic Name	Trade Name	Class and Use	Strength and Form
calcitonin	Miacalcin	polypeptide hormone	200 IU/ml spray
northindrone/ethinyl estradiol	Ortho-Novum	oral contraceptive	multiple tab
felodipine	Plendil	calcium channel blocker	2.5, 5, 10 mg tab
promethazine/codeine	Pherergan/Codeine	racemic	25, 50 mcg/ml injection
nitroglycerin	Nitroquick	vasodilator	5 mg/ml injection
spironolactone	Aldactone	aldosterone antagonist	25, 50, 100 mg tab
terazosin	Hytrin	adrenoceptor blocker	1 mg cap
finasteride	Proscar	steroid inhibitor	5 mg tab
irbesartan/HCTZ	Avalide	angiotensin receptor antagonist/diuretic	$\frac{150}{12.5}$, $\frac{300}{12.5}$ tab
desogestrel/ethinyl estradiol	Kariva	oral contraceptive	multiple tab
	Ortho-Cept-12 & 28	oral contraceptive	multiple tab
norgestrel/ethinyl estradiol	Low-Ogestrel	oral contraceptive	multiple tab
tobramycin/ dexamethasone	Tobradex	optical antibiotic/steroid	0.3 mg/ml, 0.3 mg/g suspension, ointment
mirtazapine	Remeron	tetracycline antibiotic	15, 30 mg tab
oxycodone/ acetaminophen	Roxicet	analgesic, antipyretic	$\frac{500}{5}$ mg cap
oxycodone/ acetaminophen	Percocet	analgesic, antipyretic	$\frac{500}{5}$ mg cap
ipratropium	Atrovent	anticholinergic bronchodilator	0.2% inhalant
propranolol	Inderal	beta-adrenergic blocker	10, 20, 40, 60, 80 mg tab
nifedipine	Nifediac CC	calcium channel blocker	30, 60, 90 mg tab
desogestrel/ethinyl estradiol	Apri	oral contraceptive	multiple tab

Drug Origins

Drugs are derived from five sources: plants, animals, minerals, synthesis, and bioengineering.

PLANTS

Our ancestors long ago discovered that the roots, leaves, and seeds of certain plants had the ability to cure illness, ease pain, and affect the mind. Today many drugs are still made from plant parts. A few examples are opium, belladonna, vitamin C, and digitalis.

ANIMALS

Drugs of animal origin are prepared by extracting natural substances, such as hormones, from animal tissue and organs. Insulin, for example, is extracted from the pancreas of cattle and pigs. Heparin, which is used to reduce the formation of blood clots, is taken from the intestinal linings of cattle and pigs.

MINERALS

Iron, iodine, calcium, and sodium chloride (salt) are examples of minerals used in drug therapy. They come from rocks and crystals found in nature.

SYNTHESIS

Many drugs are made in a laboratory through chemical processes. An example is omeprazole (Prilosec®), a drug used to treat GERD and other acid-related conditions.

BIOENGINEERING

Biogenetic engineering methods involve patching together DNA material from different organisms in order to produce drugs and drug products. Examples are vaccines and HGH (human growth hormone).

Drug Uses

The study of drugs will give you an understanding of drug therapy. This will be helpful as you function as a pharmacy technician in a pharmacy practice setting. Drugs are used in both healthy and sick individuals. The four most common uses of drugs are disease prevention, treatment, diagnosis, and cure. Two additional uses are contraceptives and maintenance.

Disease prevention involves the administration of drugs, such as vaccines, that inoculate the body against disease germs. Health maintenance is closely related to disease prevention. Drugs such as vitamins and insulin are given to help keep the body healthy and strong or to keep the body systems functioning normally.

Treating disease means relieving the symptoms while the body's natural disease-fighting mechanisms do their work. Aspirin and antihistamines are examples of drugs used to treat disease symptoms. Curing disease generally means eliminating disease-causing germs. Antibiotics such as penicillin are used to help cure disease.

Diagnostic drugs are prescribed to enable physicians to determine whether disease is present. For example, radiopaque dye, a dye that shows up on fluoroscope or x-rays, is administered to detect gall bladder and thyroid malfunctions.

Contraceptive drugs are used in the prevention of pregnancy. They work by controlling fertility. Drugs often have more than one use; some drugs have the ability to prevent, cure, or treat disease.

Drug Names

All drugs have more than one name, in fact, most have at least four: a chemical name, a generic name, an official name, and one or more trade names.

CHEMICAL NAME

This name describes the chemical structure of the drug. It usually is very long and complicated (Figure 6-1).

Chemical Name

AM:L27
PRESCRIBING INFORMATION

AMOXIL®
(amoxicillin capsules, tablets, chewable tablets, and powder for oral suspension)

To reduce the development of drug-resistant bacteria and maintain the effectiveness of AMOXIL (amoxicillin) and other antibacterial drugs, AMOXIL should be used only to treat or prevent infections that are proven or strongly suspected to be caused by bacteria.

DESCRIPTION

Formulations of AMOXIL contain amoxicillin, a semisynthetic antibiotic, an analog of ampicillin, with a broad spectrum of bactericidal activity against many gram-positive and gram-negative microorganisms. Chemically, it is (2S,5R,6R)-6-[(R)-(-)-2-amino-2-(p-hydroxyphenyl)acetamido]-3,3-dimethyl-7-oxo-4-thia-1-azabicyclo[3.2.0]heptane-2-carboxylic acid trihydrate. It may be represented structurally as:

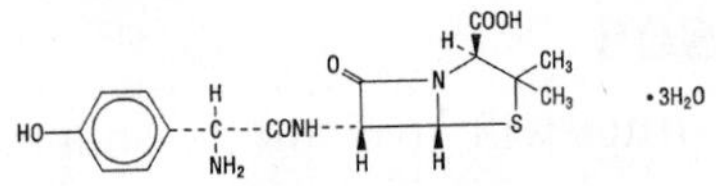

The amoxicillin molecular formula is $C_{16}H_{19}N_3O_5S \bullet 3H_2O$, and the molecular weight is 419.45.

Capsules, tablets, and powder for oral suspension of AMOXIL are intended for oral administration.

Capsules: Each capsule of AMOXIL, with royal blue opaque cap and pink opaque body, contains 500 mg amoxicillin as the trihydrate. The cap and body of the 500-mg capsule are imprinted with AMOXIL and 500. Inactive ingredients: D&C Red No. 28, FD&C Blue No. 1, FD&C Red No. 40, gelatin, magnesium stearate, and titanium dioxide.

Tablets: Each tablet contains 500 mg or 875 mg amoxicillin as the trihydrate. Each film-coated, capsule-shaped, pink tablet is debossed with AMOXIL centered over 500 or 875, respectively. The 875-mg tablet is scored on the reverse side. Inactive ingredients: Colloidal silicon dioxide, crospovidone, FD&C Red No. 30 aluminum lake, hypromellose, magnesium stearate, microcrystalline cellulose, polyethylene glycol, sodium starch glycolate, and titanium dioxide.

Chewable Tablets: Each cherry-banana-peppermint-flavored tablet contains 200 mg or 400 mg amoxicillin as the trihydrate.

Each 200-mg chewable tablet contains 0.0005 mEq (0.0107 mg) of sodium; the 400-mg chewable tablet contains 0.0009 mEq (0.0215 mg) of sodium. The 200-mg and 400-mg pale pink round tablets are imprinted with the product name AMOXIL and 200 or 400 along the edge of 1 side. Inactive ingredients: Aspartame*, crospovidone NF, FD&C Red No. 40 aluminum lake, flavorings, magnesium stearate, and mannitol.
*See PRECAUTIONS.

Figure 6-1 The chemical name of a drug (*Courtesy of GlaxoSmithKline*)

GENERIC NAME

This is the name given to a drug by the manufacturer (with input from various regulatory agencies) before the drug becomes officially recognized. It gives some information about the chemical makeup of the drug, but not as much as its chemical name (Figure 6-2). The generic name is established by the United States Adopted Names (USAN) Council. Generic is also a term used for the non-brand-name drug.

Generic Name ────

AM:L27
PRESCRIBING INFORMATION

AMOXIL®
(amoxicillin capsules, tablets, chewable tablets, and powder for oral suspension)

To reduce the development of drug-resistant bacteria and maintain the effectiveness of AMOXIL (amoxicillin) and other antibacterial drugs, AMOXIL should be used only to treat or prevent infections that are proven or strongly suspected to be caused by bacteria.

DESCRIPTION

Formulations of AMOXIL contain amoxicillin, a semisynthetic antibiotic, an analog of ampicillin, with a broad spectrum of bactericidal activity against many gram-positive and gram-negative microorganisms. Chemically, it is (2S,5R,6R)-6-[(R)-(-)-2-amino-2-(p-hydroxyphenyl)acetamido]-3,3-dimethyl-7-oxo-4-thia-1-azabicyclo[3.2.0]heptane-2-carboxylic acid trihydrate. It may be represented structurally as:

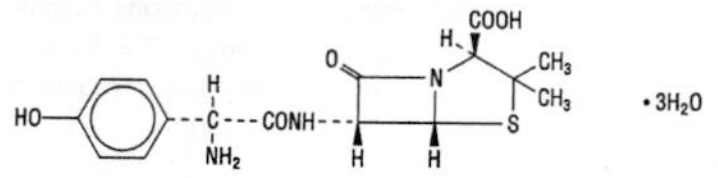

The amoxicillin molecular formula is $C_{16}H_{19}N_3O_5S \bullet 3H_2O$, and the molecular weight is 419.45.

Capsules, tablets, and powder for oral suspension of AMOXIL are intended for oral administration.
Capsules: Each capsule of AMOXIL, with royal blue opaque cap and pink opaque body, contains 500 mg amoxicillin as the trihydrate. The cap and body of the 500-mg capsule are imprinted with AMOXIL and 500. Inactive ingredients: D&C Red No. 28, FD&C Blue No. 1, FD&C Red No. 40, gelatin, magnesium stearate, and titanium dioxide.
Tablets: Each tablet contains 500 mg or 875 mg amoxicillin as the trihydrate. Each film-coated, capsule-shaped, pink tablet is debossed with AMOXIL centered over 500 or 875, respectively. The 875-mg tablet is scored on the reverse side. Inactive ingredients: Colloidal silicon dioxide, crospovidone, FD&C Red No. 30 aluminum lake, hypromellose, magnesium stearate, microcrystalline cellulose, polyethylene glycol, sodium starch glycolate, and titanium dioxide.
Chewable Tablets: Each cherry-banana-peppermint-flavored tablet contains 200 mg or 400 mg amoxicillin as the trihydrate.

Each 200-mg chewable tablet contains 0.0005 mEq (0.0107 mg) of sodium; the 400-mg chewable tablet contains 0.0009 mEq (0.0215 mg) of sodium. The 200-mg and 400-mg pale pink round tablets are imprinted with the product name AMOXIL and 200 or 400 along the edge of 1 side. Inactive ingredients: Aspartame*, crospovidone NF, FD&C Red No. 40 aluminum lake, flavorings, magnesium stearate, and mannitol.
*See PRECAUTIONS.

Figure 6-2 The generic name for a drug (*Courtesy of GlaxoSmithKline*)

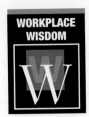
OFFICIAL NAME

This is the name under which the drug is listed in the USP/NF (United States Pharmacopeia/National Formulary). It is usually, but not always, the same as the generic name (Figure 6-3).

TRADE NAME

Also known as the brand or proprietary name, the trade name is the name under which a drug is sold by a specific manufacturer (Figure 6-4). The name is owned by the drug company, and no other company may use it. A drug manufactured by several companies may be known by several different trade names. Keep in mind, however, that although a drug may have several trade names, it can only have one generic name.

AM:L27
PRESCRIBING INFORMATION

Official Name ——

AMOXIL®
(amoxicillin capsules, tablets, chewable tablets, and powder for oral suspension)

To reduce the development of drug-resistant bacteria and maintain the effectiveness of AMOXIL (amoxicillin) and other antibacterial drugs, AMOXIL should be used only to treat or prevent infections that are proven or strongly suspected to be caused by bacteria.

DESCRIPTION

Formulations of AMOXIL contain amoxicillin, a semisynthetic antibiotic, an analog of ampicillin, with a broad spectrum of bactericidal activity against many gram-positive and gram-negative microorganisms. Chemically, it is (2S,5R,6R)-6-[(R)-(-)-2-amino-2-(p-hydroxyphenyl)acetamido]-3,3-dimethyl-7-oxo-4-thia-1-azabicyclo[3.2.0]heptane-2-carboxylic acid trihydrate. It may be represented structurally as:

The amoxicillin molecular formula is $C_{16}H_{19}N_3O_5S \cdot 3H_2O$, and the molecular weight is 419.45.

Capsules, tablets, and powder for oral suspension of AMOXIL are intended for oral administration.

Capsules: Each capsule of AMOXIL, with royal blue opaque cap and pink opaque body, contains 500 mg amoxicillin as the trihydrate. The cap and body of the 500-mg capsule are imprinted with AMOXIL and 500. Inactive ingredients: D&C Red No. 28, FD&C Blue No. 1, FD&C Red No. 40, gelatin, magnesium stearate, and titanium dioxide.

Tablets: Each tablet contains 500 mg or 875 mg amoxicillin as the trihydrate. Each film-coated, capsule-shaped, pink tablet is debossed with AMOXIL centered over 500 or 875, respectively. The 875-mg tablet is scored on the reverse side. Inactive ingredients: Colloidal silicon dioxide, crospovidone, FD&C Red No. 30 aluminum lake, hypromellose, magnesium stearate, microcrystalline cellulose, polyethylene glycol, sodium starch glycolate, and titanium dioxide.

Chewable Tablets: Each cherry-banana-peppermint-flavored tablet contains 200 mg or 400 mg amoxicillin as the trihydrate.

Each 200-mg chewable tablet contains 0.0005 mEq (0.0107 mg) of sodium; the 400-mg chewable tablet contains 0.0009 mEq (0.0215 mg) of sodium. The 200-mg and 400-mg pale pink round tablets are imprinted with the product name AMOXIL and 200 or 400 along the edge of 1 side. Inactive ingredients: Aspartame*, crospovidone NF, FD&C Red No. 40 aluminum lake, flavorings, magnesium stearate, and mannitol.

*See PRECAUTIONS.

Figure 6-3 The official name for a drug is often the same as the generic name (*Courtesy of GlaxoSmithKline*)

AM:L27
PRESCRIBING INFORMATION

Trade Name ———— AMOXIL®

(amoxicillin capsules, tablets, chewable tablets, and powder for oral
suspension)

To reduce the development of drug-resistant bacteria and maintain the effectiveness of
AMOXIL (amoxicillin) and other antibacterial drugs, AMOXIL should be used only to treat or
prevent infections that are proven or strongly suspected to be caused by bacteria.

DESCRIPTION

Formulations of AMOXIL contain amoxicillin, a semisynthetic antibiotic, an analog of
ampicillin, with a broad spectrum of bactericidal activity against many gram-positive and
gram-negative microorganisms. Chemically, it is (2S,5R,6R)-6-[(R)-(-)-2-amino-2-(p-
hydroxyphenyl)acetamido]-3,3-dimethyl-7-oxo-4-thia-1-azabicyclo[3.2.0]heptane-2-carboxylic
acid trihydrate. It may be represented structurally as:

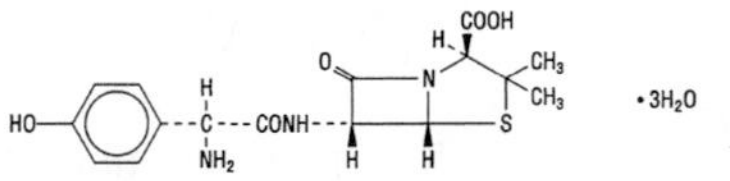

The amoxicillin molecular formula is $C_{16}H_{19}N_3O_5S \bullet 3H_2O$, and the molecular weight is
419.45.

Capsules, tablets, and powder for oral suspension of AMOXIL are intended for oral
administration.

Capsules: Each capsule of AMOXIL, with royal blue opaque cap and pink opaque body,
contains 500 mg amoxicillin as the trihydrate. The cap and body of the 500-mg capsule are
imprinted with AMOXIL and 500. Inactive ingredients: D&C Red No. 28, FD&C Blue No. 1,
FD&C Red No. 40, gelatin, magnesium stearate, and titanium dioxide.

Tablets: Each tablet contains 500 mg or 875 mg amoxicillin as the trihydrate. Each film-coated,
capsule-shaped, pink tablet is debossed with AMOXIL centered over 500 or 875, respectively.
The 875-mg tablet is scored on the reverse side. Inactive ingredients: Colloidal silicon dioxide,
crospovidone, FD&C Red No. 30 aluminum lake, hypromellose, magnesium stearate,
microcrystalline cellulose, polyethylene glycol, sodium starch glycolate, and titanium dioxide.

Chewable Tablets: Each cherry-banana-peppermint-flavored tablet contains 200 mg or
400 mg amoxicillin as the trihydrate.

Each 200-mg chewable tablet contains 0.0005 mEq (0.0107 mg) of sodium; the 400-mg
chewable tablet contains 0.0009 mEq (0.0215 mg) of sodium. The 200-mg and 400-mg pale pink
round tablets are imprinted with the product name AMOXIL and 200 or 400 along the edge of 1
side. Inactive ingredients: Aspartame*, crospovidone NF, FD&C Red No. 40 aluminum lake,
flavorings, magnesium stearate, and mannitol.

*See PRECAUTIONS.

Figure 6-4 The trade
name of a drug (*Courtesy
of GlaxoSmithKline*)

CONCLUSION

A solid understanding and knowledge of the Top 200 drugs is not only necessary for the certification exam, it is paramount to being a quality pharmacy
technician. If you have difficulty learning this information, make a set of
flash cards. Then review, review, and review.

CHAPTER REVIEW QUESTIONS

1. Which of the following drugs originates from an animal?
   a. Prilosec
   b. belladonna
   c. heparin
   d. iron

2. The official name of a drug is provided by:
   a. USP
   b. USAN
   c. the manufacturer
   d. the FDA

3. Which of the following drugs originates from a plant?
   a. Prilosec
   b. belladonna
   c. heparin
   d. iron

4. The generic name of a drug is provided by:
   a. USP
   b. USAN
   c. the manufacturer
   d. the FDA

5. Drugs are used to:
   a. cure
   b. treat
   c. diagnose
   d. all of the above

MATCHING

6. promethazine _____   a. Xanax®

7. alprazolam _____   b. Vicodin®

8. atenolol _____   c. Phenergan®

9. furosemide_____   d. Lasix®

10. hydrocodone w/APAP _____   e. Tenormin®

Community Pharmacy Operations

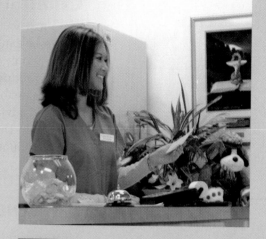

After completing this chapter, you should be able to:

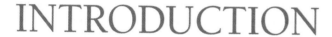

INTRODUCTION

The two main types of pharmacy practice are ambulatory and institutional. Basically, if the patient resides where the pharmacy is located, it is an institutional setting. Examples of these are hospital, nursing home, hospice, and long-term care facilities. Most other settings fall under the category of ambulatory. Examples of ambulatory settings are privately owned, chain or franchise, and clinics. Ambulatory pharmacies are also known as community or retail pharmacies, because they serve the local community in which they are located. It is well known that the community pharmacy is one of the most accessible patient health care settings available. There are a vast number of career opportunities in ambulatory pharmacies. One such opportunity is a position in a retail setting.

- Explain the ambulatory pharmacy practice setting.
- Describe the typical work environment and discuss the various positions and roles for technicians in community pharmacies.
- List and describe the two main types of community pharmacies and describe the different ways prescriptions arrive.
- List the legal requirements of a prescription medication order.
- Compare the duties of a technician with those of a pharmacist in processing and filling a prescription.
- Apply pharmacy calculations to filling a prescription correctly and list the steps required for a prescription medication order to be filled.
- Discuss the billing process for ambulatory pharmacy prescriptions.
- Demonstrate a knowledge and understanding of the insurance process and list the key components necessary for insurance billing.
- Explain the importance of good customer relations.
- List reasons why patients may have special needs and describe ways technicians can service patients.
- Discuss professionalism.

Community or Retail Pharmacy

The most well known attribute of the retail (or community) pharmacy is face-to-face interaction between the pharmacist, technicians, and the patients. Many people rely on the pharmacy team's knowledge of over-the-counter (OTC) products and prescription drugs. The retail pharmacy staff is usually more accessible to the general public than a doctor's office or clinic when it comes to advice and information on drugs.

Within the retail or community setting, ownership can differentiate the types of opportunities or tasks a technician may face.

INDEPENDENT PHARMACIES

Most independent pharmacies are privately owned, are small in size, and usually fill, on average, 100 prescriptions daily. This type of pharmacy is thought of as a neighborhood pharmacy. It generally can provide more personalized services to the customer. In this setting, the pharmacy staff can become better acquainted with its patients.

Some of the independents can provide a broader range of care than the larger chain pharmacies. This care may include preparing compounded medications, dispensing home health care products and surgical supplies, providing a delivery service, and even maintaining patient charge accounts.

Most pharmacy technicians choose a community pharmacy first because they feel that the training and experience they receive is invaluable as a foundation for future positions. Community pharmacy allows a more hands-on approach to practicing. It involves reviewing, preparing, and recording prescription orders accurately, as well as compounding some special medications. By carrying out these tasks, the pharmacy team efficiently serves and cares for its patients.

CHAIN OR FRANCHISE PHARMACIES

The other type of community pharmacy is the chain or franchise pharmacy, consisting of branches, or chains, of more than one store. Chain pharmacies generally have a higher volume (number of prescriptions), compared with the independent. Chain pharmacies are often larger and more fast paced. Chain drug stores can offer more varied career opportunities to their staffs, such as retail management and training. There is definitely room to grow within a chain pharmacy. Some will pay for the national certification exam; some offer scholarships and tuition grants for continuing education. Chain pharmacies may be in operation seven days a week and are rarely closed. In a chain pharmacy, there are usually three shifts available: morning, afternoon, and evening. Volume can differ on certain days and also during specific hours of the day.

Job Responsibilities

One of the responsibilities of a pharmacy technician in a community pharmacy is to assist the pharmacist in serving patients. The pharmacy technicians execute a variety of tasks under the supervision of the pharmacist. However, pharmacy technicians cannot counsel or give out medical information or advice to patients. It is the responsibility of the pharmacist to do this and to perform the final check before a prescription is dispensed to a patient.

Daily duties of the pharmacy technician include a vast number of jobs. Verifying drug deliveries, storing drugs, rotating stock, ordering drugs, and maintaining inventory records are just the beginning. Pharmacy technicians also verify and accept new prescription and refill orders, as well as maintain patient profiles. In addition, filling, compounding, and filing medication orders fall under the scope of the pharmacy technician's practice. Finally, technicians will assist the pharmacist in the administration of the retail pharmacy in such areas as policy and procedure review, scheduling, and formulary issues. In short, a technician will perform any task that will assist the pharmacist in serving patients or pharmacy operations, with the exception of dispensing advice or drug-related information.

Becoming a pharmacy technician in a community pharmacy setting is a very good career opportunity. Community pharmacy is a great way to establish a position of status. Customers trust the community pharmacy technician and value the services he provides. Most people who come into their local community pharmacy think of the staff as members of their families and trust the pharmacy team to provide the highest quality of service that can be given.

Processing Prescriptions

One of the first steps in providing medication for a patient is receiving the order. Remember, legend drugs may not be dispensed without a legal prescription because the government has decided that the drug has the potential for addiction or abuse or is dangerous enough to need medical supervision while being used. Pharmacy technicians are the front line in the prescription process. By reviewing an incoming prescription for legality and correctness, the technician is not only aiding the pharmacist and serving the patient, but also protecting the public.

RECEIVING THE ORDER

Most prescriptions are brought to the pharmacy by hand, but this is not the only way a prescription arrives at the pharmacy for processing. In many states, faxes are considered legal documents. It may be more convenient for a prescriber to fax the prescription directly to the pharmacy. A technician may remove faxes from the machine and fill the orders because the pharmacist

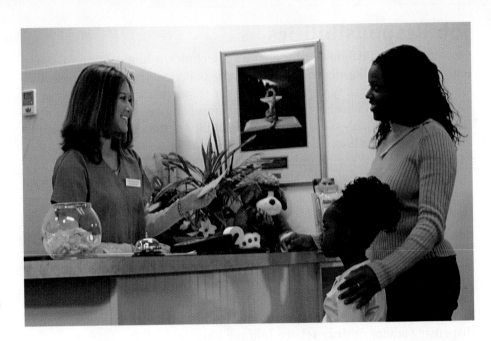

Figure 7-1 Receiving the prescription

will be reviewing and checking the orders. Most pharmacies will not give out their business fax numbers except to prescribers. If a technician is unsure of the source of a fax, he should immediately consult the pharmacist. C-II orders are the exception, because they must be handwritten, original orders and therefore cannot be faxed, e-mailed, or phoned in to the pharmacy.

Phone-in prescriptions are also very common in ambulatory practices. In most states, pharmacy technicians cannot accept a prescription by phone. As we get closer to licensing and certification to fulfill federal requirements for pharmacy technicians, this may change. But for now, when the prescriber calls in a prescription, the technician must refer the call to the pharmacist. If a patient calls in an authorized refill of an existing order, however, the technician may indeed take the order for the refill.

Computers are becoming great communication tools, and ambulatory pharmacies are no stranger to technology. Internet and mail order pharmacies, among others, may accept prescriptions via e-mail or other internet transmissions. (See Figure 7-1.)

PRESCRIPTION REQUIREMENTS

There are several pieces of information necessary before the filling process can begin. It is up to the technician to screen the orders for this information in order to save time (both the pharmacist's and patient's) and avoid waste. (See Figure 7-2.)

The first piece to this puzzle is the patient's name. It is important to get the whole name, not just a nickname. You will need to match the patient's name to the names in your patient profiles, as well as any possible insurance company records. It is the technician's responsibility to maintain current patient profiles, and this applies to name changes due to divorce or marriage.

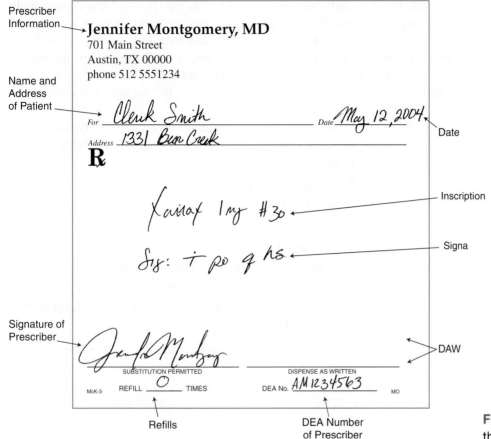

Prescriber Information — Jennifer Montgomery, MD
701 Main Street
Austin, TX 00000
phone 512 5551234

Name and Address of Patient —

For *Clenk Smith* Date *May 12, 2004* — **Date**

Address *1331 Bear Creek*

℞

Xaidax 1mg #30 — **Inscription**

Sig: ī po q hs. — **Signa**

Signature of Prescriber — *Jennifer Montgomery*

SUBSTITUTION PERMITTED   DISPENSE AS WRITTEN — **DAW**

McK-3   REFILL ___*O*___ TIMES   DEA No. *AM1234563*   MO

Refills   **DEA Number of Prescriber**

Figure 7-2 Elements of the prescription

The technician needs to verify the date the prescription was written. Remember, certain prescriptions are good for up to one year, but what about an order for an antibiotic for a child? If that prescription is being presented six months after it was written, the technician should alert the pharmacist.

Current addresses and telephone numbers are also important components of a valid prescription. This information does not have to be written on a prescription in order for the prescription to be legal, but the information has to be in the pharmacy's possession. Such information not only confirms the patient's identity, but could save his life in the event of a problem or recall.

Once the technician verifies whom the order is for, the next step is to verify the medication being ordered. The correct dosage form, strength, and quantity need to be verified. If any of these components are missing, the technician should alert the pharmacist immediately and await further instructions.

Next, the technician should review the directions for clarity and precision. Does the prescriber allow for generic substitution, or is this a DAW (dispense as written)? Are there any refills available? Remember, a C-II has no refills, a C-III can be refilled for six months, and a C-IV and a C-V may be refilled for up to a year.

Last, but certainly no less important, is the prescriber's signature. In many states, a prescriber's agent (physician's assistant or even nurse) may sign for the prescriber. Know your local laws to avoid making errors down the road. Special circumstances apply to certain medications. For instance, a C-I would most likely never be presented in an ambulatory setting. C-II prescriptions must bear no corrections or changes, be original, and contain the prescriber's DEA number.

Many errors common to ambulatory pharmacies can be avoided if the technician is knowledgeable and vigilant in accepting prescriptions. Some of the more common negative scenarios include the following:

- improper patient identification
- duplicate profiles for the same patient
- therapeutic discrepancies due to time lapse between time of prescribing and dispensing
- patient's time wasted waiting, only to find that prescription cannot be filled without further instructions from the prescriber
- inaccurate or missed insurance billing due to a lack of information or incorrect information

One of the most basic services a pharmacy technician provides to a patient, a pharmacist, or even society in general is the proper screening of prescriptions. Time, money, and even lives can be saved by performing this task efficiently and correctly. What transpires in a few moments can affect the lives of many for a lifetime.

Filling Prescriptions

Verifying a prescription order is just the beginning of the pharmacy process. Remember, you have to get the right medication in the right strength and dose to the right patient at the right time! When reduced to a system of clearly defined and followed steps, the process should run efficiently and without errors.

CHOOSING THE MEDICATION

Knowing the exact medication ordered won't help if the drug is not on your pharmacy's shelves. Inventory is a critical technician responsibility, and at this moment that fact becomes self-evident. (Assuming that the right medication is available, a few extra supply checks made at this point can save valuable time and trouble later.) The technician should check the lot number and/or the UPC numbers to ensure the medication selected is the exact medication listed on the patient's label. It is also important to check the expiration date at this point. The expiration date must not only be current the day it is dispensed, but current throughout the entire course of therapy. When selecting C-II drugs, the technician may be required to enter the medications into a log to aid in inventory control. Make sure you are aware of any state or employer policies before attempting to process a C-II prescription.

COUNTING, MEASURING, AND POURING

Counting should be done twice, until a technician feels confident in his ability. C-II prescriptions should always be counted twice before they are given to the pharmacist for a final recount. Measuring and pouring can be a little more complicated because calculations may be involved. A technician should not attempt to measure a medication until he is comfortable with the metric system as well as the household system. Consider the following prescription: The prescriber ordered Amoxil 250 mg TID × 10D. The medication is available as 125 mg/5 ml. The technician not only has to understand mg and ml, but also TID and 10D. The correct amount to be dispensed is 300 ml. (See Figure 7-3.)

LABELING

As simple as it sounds, labeling still requires attention to detail. First, the label must go onto the correct medication container. This may sound facetious, but in an assembly-line type pharmacy, many errors occur over just this detail! For technicians, this is the last chance to check your work before submitting it to the pharmacist for a final check. Double check the directions and drug strength, and affix any auxiliary labels that may be appropriate. The drug label is usually generated by computer and will contain all the information required by law. Just for a quick review, that means the name and phone number of the dispensing pharmacy, the patient's name, prescription number, date, medication, strength, directions, and the name of the prescriber. The label will also show the quantity of medication inside as well as the number of refills.

FINAL CHECK

The final check is the sole domain of the pharmacist. No medications may be dispensed without the pharmacist's final approval. In an ambulatory setting, this is a relatively simple process. The pharmacist will need the original prescription and the labeled container filled with the prescribed medication. Once the pharmacist gives his OK, the medication may be given to the patient.

Insurance Billing

We hear almost every day about the high cost of health care. Prescription costs are a contributing factor in that equation. To help defray the cost of prescriptions, many Americans have individually purchased or employer-subsidized prescription insurance. One of the responsibilities of an ambulatory pharmacy technician is to process insurance claims for patients. A few basic points to remember, coupled with some computer experience, will set the technician on the way to competence.

UNDERSTANDING THE PROCESS

Most ambulatory pharmacies bill their patient's insurance for them. The responsibility for collecting, maintaining, and transmitting insurance claims rests on the shoulders of the pharmacy technician. The entire process is usually

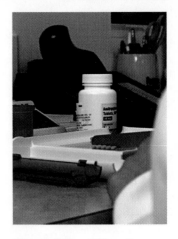

Figure 7-3 Filling the prescription

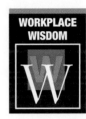

WORKPLACE WISDOM

A helpful hint for pouring medications is to always use the container size closest to the amount you are dispensing, without going under. For example, you would not pour 50 ml into a 180 ml bottle if there is a 60 ml container available.

done by computer. Through the Internet, the pharmacy electronically submits a claim to the insurance provider's computer or a third-party claims processor, and hopefully there is an exchange of funds. This exchange takes mere moments in most cases, and the patient is on his way.

INSURANCE TERMS

Just as in the pharmacy setting, the insurance world has its own set of terms used in conducting its business. Following are some of the more common ones:

- Carrier/Insurer/Provider—the insurance company
- Processor—a company hired by the insurer to process claims
- Claim—a request for reimbursement from a health care provider to an insurance provider for products or services rendered
- Co-pay—a portion of the cost of a service or product that a patient pays out of pocket each time it is provided. For example, Mrs. Brown pays $5 for each prescription regardless of the cost of the medication
- Deductible—a set amount that a client pays up front before insurance coverage applies. This may be paid at once or in parts. For example, Mrs. Brown has a $100 deductible. Her insurer may pay only 80 percent of each claim until she has paid $100 and then her carrier pays 100 percent
- DAW "Dispense as Written"—used by prescribers to instruct the pharmacy to use the exact drug written (usually brand). Insurance providers may request the prescriber to state, in writing, his medical reasoning behind such a choice
- Days Supply—the number of days a dispensed quantity of medication will last

COLLECTING DATA

Just as the pharmacy keeps a confidential patient profile on all the clients it serves, insurance providers, public or private, do likewise. (See Figure 7-4.) When a third party is hired by an insurance provider to process claims, the client information is provided by the insurer to the adjustors. Whether it be the government (Medicaid and Medicare) or a private insurer (Blue Cross®, Aetna®, etc.), all providers keep records on their customers. These records contain much of the same information as the pharmacy patient profile.

Before a claim can be paid, the information has to match exactly on both sides of the Internet. Starting with the correct name, the insurer will also provide an account number and possibly a personal code. Marriages, divorces, and births all can affect the continuation of insurance coverage. It is the technician's responsibility to collect all the current relevant information required for insurance billing for the pharmacy, but it is the patient's responsibility to keep the insurance provider's information updated.

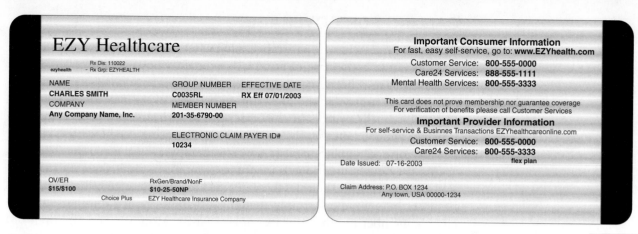

Figure 7-4   Sample insurance card

An example of this process would be as follows: When Mary Smith was married, she changed her name to Brown. The new Mrs. Brown dutifully changed her credit cards, address, and driver's license information. When she came to the pharmacy, the astute technician also updated her profile in the computer. However, when her insurance claim was submitted, it was refused! Why? Because Mrs. Brown had neglected to update her records with her insurance provider, the information submitted by the pharmacy, although correct, did not match the information in the insurance provider's records. The claim was denied. Therefore, even when all pharmacy records are accurate in order for insurance billing to work, the two profiles (pharmacy and insurance) must match exactly.

THE PRESCRIPTION

Assuming that the patient profiles match, a billing pharmacy technician is just getting started. The insurance provider will need to know the name of the medication being dispensed. Providers, just like pharmacies, have formularies. In other words, the insurance provider will pay only for approved medications. Along with the strength and dose, there is the question of brand or generic.

Providers will usually pay much more of the cost of a generic medication and defer more of the cost of a brand drug back to the patient. The magic exception here is the DAW code that may be provided by a doctor for medical reasons. Note the following example: Mrs. Brown requested that a brand-name drug be used in filling her prescription. Her normal co-pay is $5, but this time the claim came back, charging $72. The reason is that Mrs. Brown's insurance will not pay for a brand-name drug unless her doctor claims that it is medically necessary by writing "DAW" on her prescription.

If a technician places the DAW there in error, he could be charged with insurance fraud. If Mrs. Brown did not request brand, but the prescriber did, and the technician forgot to put "DAW" in the claim, Mrs. Brown may end up paying way too much.

CALLING FOR COVERAGE

There are times when an insurance issue cannot be handled by computer. A good example is the case of an elderly woman whose doctor ordered birth control pills as a hormone replacement. The insurance computer automatically refused to pay for the prescription because of the provider's policy not to pay for birth control. In this case, the technician may need to call the provider and explain that the medication is not being used for birth control, but for hormone replacement (a covered therapy).

As previously mentioned, insurance computers simply match information coming in with their database. Twins are an insurance billing challenge because the computers simply match the parent's policy number with the eligible member number (for example, Dad-01, Mom-02, and Children-03) and birth dates. Unfortunately, twins have the exact same birth dates. If they are both to receive a prescription, the provider may have to be contacted by phone before the proper payment can be made.

COMMON BILLING ERRORS

- Incorrect name: may be due to nicknames, marriage, or divorce
- Incorrect days supply: will affect refill times and insurance reimbursements
- Incorrect provider: due to changes in employment or employer benefits
- Incorrect birth date: can be entered incorrectly for a number of reasons

The preceding errors will cause the following refusal messages:

- "Patient not covered": could be incorrect name, birth date, incorrect provider, or new coverage
- "Too early to refill": could be the wrong days supply was entered

A technician should never take these types of messages at face value, but rather continue investigating. This is part of good patient service. There are times, however, when you have done all you can do to effect a payment from a provider on behalf of your patient.

Insurance billing is a wonderful customer service that pharmacy technicians provide for their patients each day. Insurance billing is done electronically. When machines talk to machines, they communicate only as well as the people operating them. Human intervention can save the day and humanize what can be a very cold process.

Customer Service

Many pages have now been devoted to discussing the importance of providing the right patient with the right medication, and so on, but there is more to the practice of pharmacy than counting, typing, and measuring. In the whirlwind of activity called "medication dispensing," it is imperative that we do not forget the patient!

FOCUS ON THE PATIENT

As technicians, we have so many different responsibilities, it becomes easy to "miss the forest for the trees." The focus is, and will always be, on the patient. Patients need and deserve a lot more from us than medication. So, take a closer look. What are some qualities or characteristics of a typical patient? First, they are seeking medication. This should tell you that they are feeling less than 100 percent well or are assisting someone in that situation. Patients may also be afraid. For some people, not being in control is very frightening, and fear of the future can be very real. Patients are often stressed, in pain, or experiencing discomfort. All of the aforementioned conditions can cloud a person's judgment and most certainly alter their personalities. In short, patients are often not themselves. As health care professionals, this is what technicians have to work with. There is a lot you can do to help if you care enough. (See Figure 7-5.)

PATIENT NEEDS

Anyone being waited on, whether at a cash register or a doctor's office, wants attention. Not to acknowledge a customer is an insult, no matter how busy you may be. A smile and a nod goes a long way and takes little time or effort.

Everyone likes to feel important, including your patients. They may not realize that the very reason you cannot chat with them is that you are working to ensure their own safety. Often, it is not so much what you do, but how you do it. Everyone wants to be understood. Sometimes, you may become frustrated when you reach the end of what you can do, and your patient is still not satisfied; but ask yourself, "Have I expressed my understanding?" Starting your next sentence with "I understand how frustrating this is for you, but..." at least shows that you care.

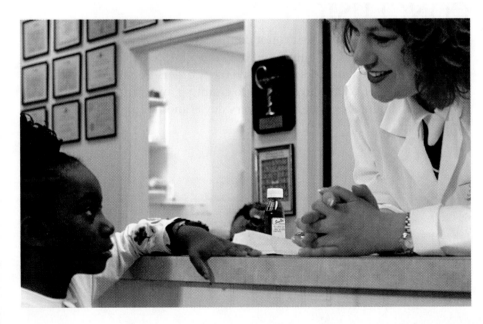

Figure 7-5 Focusing on the patient

Validation is also something everyone craves. It is okay to be frustrated or angry when things do not go right. Technicians should not be afraid to recognize this in patients. Because you understand their frustration and agree with their outrage does not mean that you can do anything about the situation; but it does show that you care, and this validates their feelings.

A pharmacist's time is valuable. The pharmacist certainly does not have time to do something over because the technician either did it wrong or, as in the following example, not well enough. The pharmacist should not have to re-explain to Mrs. Brown

- why her medication was not ordered in sufficient quantity to be filled today,
- why the price went up or why her refill cannot be done today, or
- why her insurance will not pay for her prescription.

If you handle the situation properly, you not only can save the pharmacist time, but also can take better care of Mrs. Brown.

Of course, there will be situations that are simply impossible, and certainly the pharmacist is there to help, but often it just takes the proper attitude and a little effort to make things right.

PROFESSIONALISM

When it comes to patient service, professionalism is your sharpest tool. Think of professionalism as a suit of armor that protects you from acting out or taking negativism personally. Professionalism is an attitude, a code of actions, and a standard of ethics all rolled into one. By developing a sense of professionalism, you can get through difficult situations, show compassion, and maintain your sanity while remaining effective and accurate.

CONCLUSION

While pharmacy technicians cannot counsel people, they can certainly take care of patients' insurance billing and help them locate OTC medications and their prices. Technicians take care of inventory orders, rotations, returns, and billings. This is, of course, in addition to counting, measuring, filling, and labeling. In an ambulatory pharmacy, every day is another opportunity to serve the community.

PROFILES

OF PRACTICE

Can you decipher the sample prescriptions in Figures 7-6 through 7-8?

What is wrong with the prescriptions in Figure 7-9 and Figure 7-10?

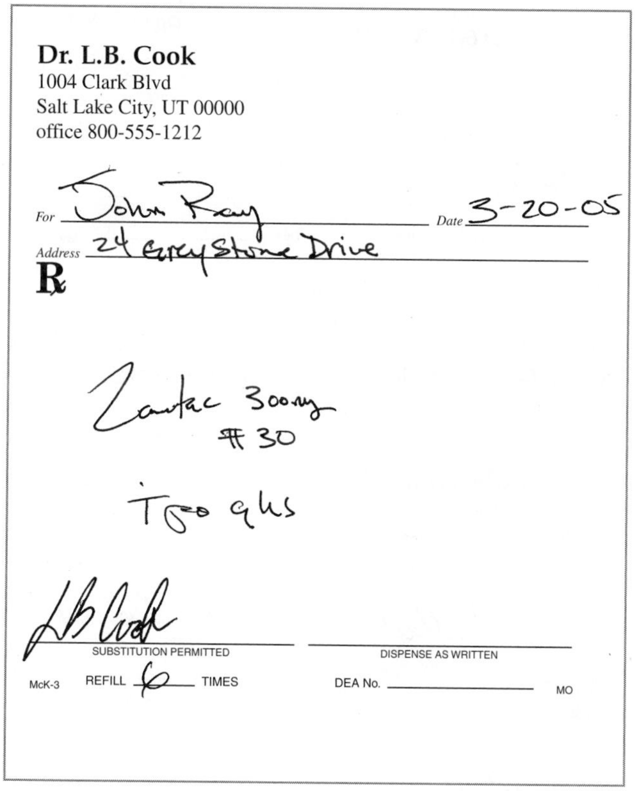

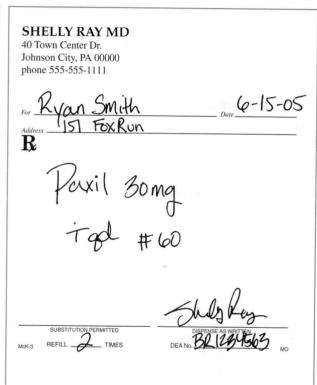

Dr. L.B. Cook
1004 Clark Blvd
Salt Lake City, UT 00000
office 800-555-1212

For John Ray   Date 3-20-05
Address 24 Greystone Drive

R

Zantac 300mg
30

T̄ qhs

LB Cook
SUBSTITUTION PERMITTED   DISPENSE AS WRITTEN
McK-3   REFILL 6 TIMES   DEA No. _____ MO

Figure 7-6 Sample prescription

SHELLY RAY MD
40 Town Center Dr.
Johnson City, PA 00000
phone 555-555-1111

For Ryan Smith   Date 6-15-05
Address 151 FoxRun

R

Paxil 30mg
T̄ qd #60

Shelly Ray
SUBSTITUTION PERMITTED   DISPENSE AS WRITTEN
McK-3   REFILL 2 TIMES   DEA No. BR1234563 MO

Figure 7-7 Sample prescription

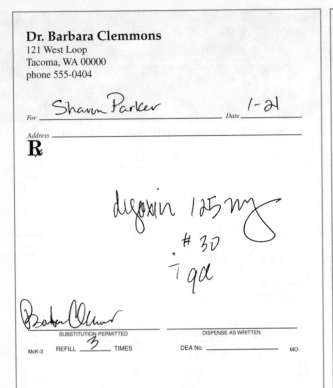

Figure 7-8   Sample prescription

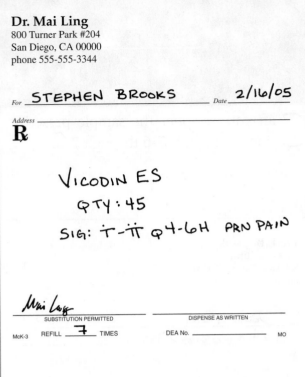

Figure 7-9   Sample prescription with error(s)

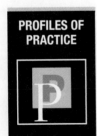

PROFILES OF PRACTICE

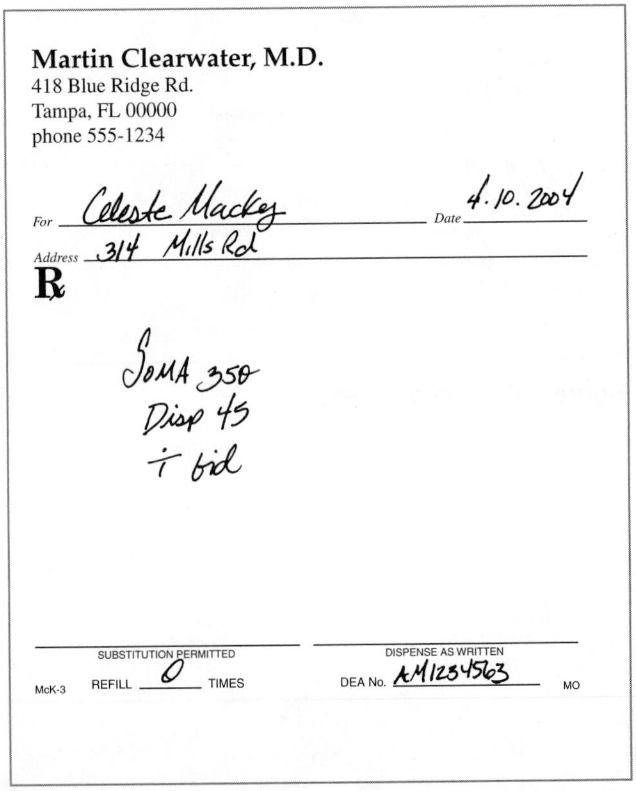

Figure 7-10   Sample prescription with error(s)

CHAPTER REVIEW QUESTIONS

1. Which of the following is not an example of ambulatory or retail pharmacy?
   a. franchise or chain pharmacy
   b. nursing home pharmacy
   c. privately owned pharmacy
   d. All of the above are examples.

2. The term "ambulatory pharmacy" refers to a setting in which:
   a. the patient arrives by ambulance.
   b. the patient lives at the facility where the pharmacy is located.
   c. the patient walks into the pharmacy.
   d. the pharmacy is part of a larger facility.

3. Which of the following does not need to be recorded on a prescription?
   a. prescriber's signature
   b. patient's age
   c. medication quantity and strength
   d. patient's complete name

4. The proper prescription needs to contain which of the following drug information?
   a. name of the medication
   b. strength
   c. dosage form
   d. all of the above

5. Which of the following is not the responsibility of a technician?
   a. verifying patient's name, address, and phone number
   b. checking for drug name, quantity, strength, dose, and route
   c. verifying the final prescription
   d. entering the insurance information and billing the provider

6. Which of the following tasks may a technician not perform?
   a. fill a prescription from a fax
   b. accept a refill order from a patient
   c. accept a prescription order by phone
   d. call an insurer on behalf of a patient

7. Before selecting the medication to fill an order, a technician should:
   a. check the brand name
   b. check the NDC and/or UPC code
   c. check the contraindications
   d. check with the pharmacist

8. Which of the following does not appear on the patient's bottle?
   a. name of the medication being dispensed
   b. quantity of the medication being dispensed
   c. phone number of the prescriber
   d. phone number of the pharmacy

9. A co-pay is:
   a. when a third party pays part of the cost of medication
   b. what an insurer pays toward the cost of medication.
   c. the portion of the cost the pharmacy can bill the patient for later
   d. the portion of the cost of a prescription a patient pays each time

10. A deductible is:
    a. the profit margin a pharmacy gets to keep
    b. what a patient pays each time they get a prescription filled
    c. a set fee paid out of pocket before any or full benefits are paid
    d. all of the above

Resources and References

1. Reifman, Noah. *Certification Review for Pharmacy Technicians, 6th Ed.* Evergreen, CO: Ark Pharmaceutical Consultants, Inc., 2002.

2. American Pharmacist Association. *Pharmacy Technician Workbook and Certification Review.* Englewood, CO: Morton Publishing, 2001.

3. American Society of Health System Pharmacists. *Manual for Pharmacy Technicians.* Bethesda, MD: ASHP, 1998.

4. American Society of Health System Pharmacists. *Pharmacy Technician Certification Review and Exam.* Bethesda, MD: ASHP, 1998.

5. Ballington, Don. *Pharmacy Practice.* St. Paul, MN: EMC Paradigm, 1999.

6. Ballington, Don. *Pharmacy Practice for Technicians.* St. Paul, MN: EMC Paradigm, 2003.

7. Cowen, D. and W. Helfand. *Pharmacy: An Illustrated History.* New York: Harry N. Abrams, Incorporated, 1990.

8. Lambert, Anita. *Advanced Pharmacy Practice for Technicians.* Clifton Park, NY: Delmar, 2002.

9. Ansel, H.C., *Introduction to Pharmaceutical Dosage Forms.* Philadelphia: Lea & Febiger, 1995.

10. The American Medical Association. *Know Your Drugs and Medications.* New York, NY: The Reader's Digest Association, 1991.

11. Facts and Comparisons. "Homepage." January 2004. *http://www.factsandcomparisons.com*

12. Food and Drug Administration. "Homepage." January 2004. *http://www.fda.gov*

Community Pharmacy Calculations

VICODIN ES
   QTY: 45
SIG: ī-īī Q4-6H   PRN PAIN

INTRODUCTION

The various mathematical equations and formulas used by pharmacy technicians in the community-based pharmacy are similar to those required of a technician working in an institution, with some obvious exceptions. This chapter concerns those calculations, manipulations, and other matters that you need to master before you can correctly fill a prescription.

Learning Objectives

After completing this chapter, you should be able to:

- Describe and use the metric system of measurements.
- Perform dosage calculations.
- Accurately determine temperature conversions.
- Calculate advanced alligation-based problems.

Note: This chapter does not cover basic math principles.
For a more in-depth review, refer to Pharmacy Calculations in
the Pharmacy Technician Series, published by Prentice Hall Health.

Background to Community Pharmacy Calculations

There is obviously a great deal of overlap in the duties and responsibilities of the pharmacy technician working in a community pharmacy and the technician working in an institution such as an acute care facility.

Regardless of the differences between the two settings, every pharmacy technician ought to become familiar with the duties and responsibilities of both. One day he may find himself working in a community pharmacy that has obtained a contract to fill medications for a long-term care facility.

While it is true that, due to the vast array of recent technological advancements, many of the older apothecary calculations are no longer needed, it is also true that there remain a good number of medications that require attention to detail with respect to mathematics before the prescription can be correctly filled.

The Metric System

The metric system needs to be well mastered in all aspects of pharmacy work. The metric system is, in fact, the preferred method used in all pharmacies because it is easier to work with and is more accurate than the household measurement system. You will need to master the conversions,* especially with respect to weight and volume, shown as follows:

1 kilogram = 1000 grams

1 gram = 1000 milligrams

1 milligram = 1000 micrograms (μg)

1 liter = 1000 milliliters, or 1000 cubic centimeters, or approximately 1 quart

480 ml = approximately 1 pint

240 ml = approximately 8 fluid ounces

30 ml = approximately 1 fluid ounce

1 ml = 1cc

Dosage Calculations

Perhaps one of the more common computation problems for the pharmacy technician is the dosage calculation. Determine the number of doses, the quantity of each dose, or the size of each dose to be dispensed by using the following formula:

• Number of doses = Total quantity divided by the size of each dose

---

*Expanded charts on systems of measurement are included in Appendix B of this book.

EXAMPLE 8.1 How many doses would be contained in 2 grams of a medication if the dosage is 50 mg? (In other words, if you have 2 grams of the medication and the patient is to take 50 mg of the medication, how many doses are available in that quantity?)

- Number of Doses = 2000 mg (convert the grams to milligrams) divided by 50 mg
- Therefore, the number of doses in this quantity is 40.

Now look at this problem from a different angle. If you have a prescription that calls for 30 grams, divided into 20 doses, what size doses should be administered?

- Begin by setting up the problem:

  20 doses = 30 gm divided by x (the unknown)

  $20x = 30$ grams (Here, manipulate the formula without changing the value of the equation; that is, cross multiply—there is an imaginary '1' under the 20.)

  $x = 1.5$ grams per dose (Here, perform a little bit of algebra by dividing both sides of the equation by 20, which does not change the value of the formula. Remember that you can do anything to an equation as long as you do the same to both sides of the equation; the point is to get x on one side of the equation.)

EXAMPLE 8.2 You are tasked with calculating the amount of syrup that is to be dispensed to provide 20 doses, that is, four times a day, or QID of 5 ml per dose of a specific medication.

- Set up the formula: $20/1 = x/5$ ml (Here, you have another proportion.)
- $x = 100$ ml. How did you get that answer? Easy. Cross multiply and eliminate the number in front of the x—again, the point is to get x—the variable—by itself.

EXAMPLE 8.3 Suppose a patient brings in a prescription written by a physician or physician assistant for the following medication and written in the following way: Amoxil, 250 mg/5 ml, Sig: 1 teaspoon po tid for 10 days.

How much of the liquid medication should you dispense?

You need to know the quantity of the medication to be dispensed, correct? In other words, your job would be to calculate the total volume needed: To calculate this, simply multiply 3(5 ml) × 10 days, which equals:
$15 \times 3 \times 10 = 45 \times 10 = 150$ ml.

Pediatric Dosage Calculations

There are four different methods used to compute the doses for children: Young's Rule, Clark's Rule, Fried's Rule, and Body Surface Area Rule. Dosing for the pediatric population is based on age, body surface area, and, finally, the weight of the child.

- Young's Rule:
  [age of child/(age of child + 12)] × adult dose = child's dose

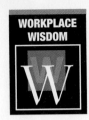
In contemporary practice, the most widely accepted method of calculating pediatric dosages is mg/kg/day, in which you simply multiply the child's weight (in kg) by the manufacturer's recommended dosage in mg per kg daily.

- Clark's Rule: weight of child/150 lb × adult dose = child's dose
- Fried's Rule:
  age in months/150 × average adult dose = child's dose
- Body Surface Area Rule: body surface of child
  (square meters)/1.7 × adult dose = child's dose

EXAMPLE 8.4   A three-year-old girl weighs approximately 30 pounds. Her mother approaches the pharmacist with the following question: "How much cough syrup should I give my child?" The bottle has been in the house for some time, and the label has worn off, but the mother does not want to buy another bottle. She knows that the adult dose is 2 teaspoons every 4 hours. The pharmacist asks you to figure the dose while he takes a phone call from a doctor. How much medicine should the woman give her daughter?

- Young's Rule: $\frac{3}{3}$ + 12 × 10 ml = child's dose,
  $\frac{1}{5}$ × 10 ml = 2 ml (1 teaspoon equals 5 ml, so the mother should give the child just under one half of a teaspoon, or resort to calibrated tool.)
- Clark's Rule: $\frac{30}{150}$ × 10 ml = child's dose $-\frac{1}{5}$ × 10 ml = 2 ml
- Fried's Rule: $\frac{36}{150}$ × 10 ml = child's dose, or 0.24 × 10 ml
  = 2.4 ml

Some doses are administered on a body weight basis, and therefore it is important to know how to make these conversions. Recall that 1 kilogram = 2.2 pounds. The dose, then, is multiplied by the number of the kilograms.

Temperature Conversions

There will be a number of instances while performing your functions as a pharmacy technician in which you will need to convert Fahrenheit (the American System) to Centigrade (which is typically used by most other countries). You must be able to make these conversions, because there could be some instances when the Fahrenheit system will be of no use to you.

- Centigrade: This system is calibrated so that the freezing point of water is 0 degrees and the boiling point is 100 degrees.
- Fahrenheit: In this system, the freezing point of water is 32 degrees and the boiling point is 212 degrees.

To convert from one scale to the other scale, the following formula is used:

$$9 \times C \text{ degrees} = (5 \times F \text{ degrees}) - 160$$

EXAMPLE 8.5   To convert 10 degrees C to F, the following formula is used:

- 9 × 10 = 5 F − 160 or 90 = 5 F − 160 = +160 or
  250 = 5 F, or F = 50; therefore, when C is 10 degrees,
  F is 50.

EXAMPLE 8.6   To convert 80 degrees F to C, use the same method:

- $9 \times C = (5 \times 80) - 160$
- $9\,C = 240$
- $C = 26.6$

Alligations

There will be many times during your career as a pharmacy technician when the appropriate dose of a specific medication is not available. For example, if a specific or desired percentage concentration of a solution, an ointment, or a cream is not readily available, the needed compound can easily be created with a little bit of imagination mixed with know-how. All you need to create the desired product are the elements that make up the solution, the ointment or the cream, and the know-how to add or subtract an element. And, like most other situations in pharmacy work, knowing where to start, what to add, and what not to add, is the key to such a challenge. This method, usually called an alligation alternative, is one way that you will be able to deliver an item that once did not exist in your pharmacy. Alligation is a method used to determine the desired percentage concentration of a solution, an ointment, or a cream that you need to fill for a customer when such a concentration does not already exist in your pharmacy.

EXAMPLE 8.7   What quantity of a 70 percent solution must be mixed with a 20 percent dextrose solution to obtain 1 liter (1000 ml) of a 35 percent dextrose solution?

Alligation Grid

- Write in the higher beginning strength in the top left box and the lower beginning strength in the lower left box.
- Write the desired strength in the middle box.
- Take the difference on the diagonal from lower left to upper right, and write in the upper right box.

     35 from 70 = 35. This is how many parts of the 70% solution are needed.

When figuring the difference on the diagonal, always write down a positive number.

- Take the difference on the diagonal from the upper left box to the lower right box, and write in the lower right box.

20 from 35 = 15.   This is how many parts of
the 20% are needed.

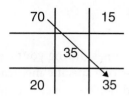

- Next, add up the third column.

15 + 35 = 50

The total of the third column is how many total parts are needed for the preparation (50 total parts).

$$
\begin{array}{c|c}
70 & 15 \\
\hline
& 35 \\
\hline
20 & 35 \\
\end{array}
$$

What we know so far is that there are a total of 50 parts.
15 parts of the total will be the 70%, and
35 parts of the total will be the 20% solution.

- Next, write out the fractions of the total. This is how many parts there are of the first percent strength over the total parts. Following along the top row of numbers, representing the 70% solution, write out the fraction of parts over the total parts. This is the number in the top right box over the total of the third column.

15 parts/50 parts

- Then, for the lower row of numbers representing the 20% solution, write out the fraction over the total. This is how many parts there are of the 20% over the total parts. This is the number in the lower right box over the total of the third column.

35 parts/50 parts

- Next, multiply each of these by the total volume you wish to prepare, which is 1000 ml.
Representing the 70%, the top row, calculate the following:

$$
\frac{15}{50} \times 1000 \text{ ml} = 300 \text{ ml}
$$

Representing the 20% on the lower row, calculate the following:

$$
\frac{35}{50} \times 1000 \text{ ml} = 700 \text{ ml}
$$

This problem looks like this across the page:

$\frac{15}{50} \times 1000$ ml $= 300$ of the 70% solution needed.

$\frac{35}{50} \times 1000$ ml $= 700$ of the 20% solution needed.

Notice that $300 + 700 = 1000$ ml. This is a quick check.

Another means of doing the same process is given in Example 8.8.

EXAMPLE 8.8   When 5 ml of 2 percent alcohol are mixed with 10 ml of 4 percent alcohol, it can be determined, through alligation, that we will obtain 15 ml of 3.33 percent alcohol. The following steps are used in this process:

Step 1: Add the quantity of each component used in the mixture.

Step 2: Multiply the quantity of each component used in the mixture by its corresponding percentage strength, and then add up the products.

Step 3: Divide the value obtained in step 2 by the value in step 1.

The same problem can be demonstrated in the following manner:

Percentages of ETOH in the mixture:

Alcohol 2% → 5 mL

Alcohol 4% → 10 mL

Step 1: $5 + 10 = 15$ mL

Step 2: $5 \times 2\% = 10$

$10 \times 4\% = 40$

Total: 50

Step 3: $\frac{50}{15} = 3.33\%$

Accounting Formulas

Selling Price = Cost + Markup

Markup = Selling Price − Cost

Markup Percent = $\dfrac{(\text{Selling price} - \text{Cost})}{\text{Cost}} \times 100$

Gross Profit = Selling Price − Invoice Cost

Gross Profit Percent = $\dfrac{(\text{Price} - \text{Cost})}{\text{Cost}} \times 100$

Net Profit = Selling Price − Cost − Overhead

CONCLUSION

As you already know, you will need to master a number of different forms of calculations in order to function correctly as a pharmacy technician, particularly now, as the pharmacy technician is being asked to perform more tasks than ever before. The more you know about taking care of a patient's prescriptions, the better you can serve the patient, the pharmacist, and the company for which you are responsible.

PRACTICE PROBLEMS

Acetaminophen Infant Pain Reliever 80 mg/0.8 ml in a 30 ml container. Dosing guideline for infants up to 3 months, 40 mg up to 5 times per day. Acquisition cost = $1.29 Markup 35%

1. Calculate the selling price. _____

2. Calculate the markup. _____

3. How many doses are contained in the dispensing package?
   _____

4. What is the dose in milligrams? _____

5. How many grams of active ingredient are contained in the dispensing package? _____

6. Rx   Progesterone 4% in Vanishing Cream 180 g
   How much active ingredient should be weighed? _____

7. Rx   Testosterone Cypionate 100 mg/ml   10 ml
   How many active ingredient should be weighed? _____

Rx   Penicillin 250 mg/5 ml   200 ml
     1 tsp qid
     Acquisition cost = $1.10
     Selling price = $8.95

8. How many days will the prescription last? _____

9. Calculate the gross profit. _____

10. Calculate the gross profit percent. _____

CHAPTER REVIEW QUESTIONS

1. This rule is used for dosing in pharmacy and based on the patient's age.
   - **a.** Andrew's Rule
   - **b.** Young's Rule
   - **c.** Mike's Rule
   - **d.** none of the above

2. 32 degrees Fahrenheit equals what degree Centigrade?
   - **a.** 10
   - **b.** 0
   - **c.** 15
   - **d.** 20

3. Using alligation, if you need 120 gm of a 40% cream and all you have available are 50% and 10%, what ratio of each do you need?
   - **a.** 1:3
   - **b.** 3:4
   - **c.** 1:5
   - **d.** 1:12

4. Calculate net profit. Diabetic Testing Strips #100, Cost = $67.00, Price = $89.79, Overhead = $4.50.
   - **a.** $22.79
   - **b.** $18.29
   - **c.** $27.29
   - **d.** $29.79

5. How many tablets should be dispensed?

   Rx   Prednisone 5 mg tablets qs

   50 mg for 2 days

   40 mg for 2 days

   35 mg for 2 days

   30 mg for 1 day

   25 mg for 1 day

   20 mg for 1 day

   10 mg for 1 day

   5 mg for 2 days

   Then stop.
   - **a.** 42 tablets
   - **b.** 50 tablets
   - **c.** 88 tablets
   - **d.** 69 tablets

6. How many milliliters are required to deliver the dose?

   Insulin 100 units/ml Dose = 20 units qam
   - **a.** 0.2 ml
   - **b.** 0.25 ml
   - **c.** 0.3 ml
   - **d.** 0.4 ml

7. Rx   Amoxicillin/Potassium Clavuante 45 mg/kg/day q12h

   Your patient is 6 years old and weighs 68 pounds.

   What is the patient's weight in kilograms?
   - **a.** 11.33 kg
   - **b.** 20.3 kg
   - **c.** 30.9 kg
   - **d.** 45 kg

8. Rx   Amoxicillin/Potassium Clavuante 45 mg/kg/day q12h

   Your patient is 6 years old and weighs 68 pounds.

   What is the total dosage per day?
   - **a.** 3060 mg
   - **b.** 1530 mg
   - **c.** 255 mg
   - **d.** 1390 mg

9. Rx   Amoxicillin/Potassium Clavuante 45 mg/kg/day q12h

   Your patient is 6 years old and weighs 68 pounds.

   How much is each dose?
   - **a.** 695 mg
   - **b.** 255 mg
   - **c.** 325 mg
   - **d.** 750 mg

10. Using the formula AWP − 14% + $2.50, what is the gross profit percent for 30 tablets of a product that has an AWP of $87.00/C and an invoice cost of $62.34/C? (C = roman numeral for 100.)
    - **a.** 18.70%
    - **b.** 33.42%
    - **c.** 24.95%
    - **d.** 6.25%

Resources and References

1. Reifman, Noah. *Certification Review for Pharmacy Technicians, 6th Ed.* Evergreen, CO: Ark Pharmaceutical Consultants, 2002.

2. Reddy, Indra and Mansoor Khan. *Essential Math and Calculations for Pharmacy Technicians.* Boca Raton, FL, and other cities: CRC Press, 2004.

Introduction to Compounding

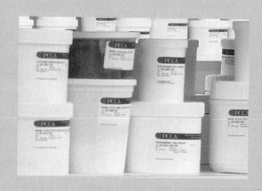

INTRODUCTION

Webster's New World Dictionary defines the word compound as a verb meaning "1. to mix or combine, 2. to make by combining parts, and 3. to intensify by adding new elements." Pharmaceutical compounding is the practice of extemporaneously preparing medications to meet the unique need of an individual patient according to the specific order of a prescriber. This differs from the traditional practice of pharmacy in that it involves a special relationship between patient, prescriber, and pharmacist.

Overview of Compounding

Pharmacy is the only profession that allows the extemporaneous compounding of chemicals for therapeutic care. There has been an increase in the need for compounding prescriptions. Several reasons for this increase include the discontinuation of certain drugs by their manufacturer, the removal from the market of drugs by the Food and Drug Administration, and the unavailability of drugs in a strength or dosage form appropriate for a specific patient. Patients with sensitivities or allergies to preservatives or other certain excipients will need to have their medications compounded, leaving out the offending agent(s). A combination therapy that a prescriber desires, but that is not currently commercially available, can also be successfully compounded. These are just a few of the many scenarios that require the expertise of a compounding pharmacist.

The level of difficulty of preparing the compounded prescription is determined by the physical properties of the drug being prescribed and the dosage form desired either by the prescriber or the patient. In some cases compounding will be a simple two-step process, whereas in others it will require extensive knowledge and many steps to perform.

Regardless of the procedure, certain criteria must be considered for all compounded prescriptions. Research must be done on the active ingredient to determine cost effectiveness, availability, solubility, stability, and possible dosage forms. Every pharmacy that compounds prescriptions should have access to quality reference resources. Some of these valuable resources include the following books and journals:

- *Remington's Pharmaceutical Sciences*
- *The Merck Manual*
- *The Merck Veterinary Manual*
- *Trissel's Stability of Compounded Formulations*
- *Drug Facts and Comparisons*
- *United States Pharmacopeia*
- *Veterinary Drug Handbook* by Donald C. Plumb
- *International Journal of Compounding Pharmacists*
- Various Internet websites

Compounding a Prescription

In addition to researching the active ingredients and excipients needed in a compounded prescription, the preparer must also have knowledge regarding pharmaceutical calculations. This is one area of compounding where the potential for error is great. Something as simple as a misplaced decimal point can have devastating results for the patient. Only a properly trained individual should perform the critical calculations involved in formulating a compounded prescription, and no calculation or measurement should go unchecked by the pharmacist.

The first step in compounding a prescription is to obtain a formula or recipe that is prepared by a pharmacist, including all necessary ingredients and explicit instructions for the preparer. The source of the formula may be one that has already been published or that has been created by the pharmacist in the compounding facility. If a formula is handwritten, it must be written legibly, with instructions communicated clearly to the preparer. From the formula or recipe, a worksheet should be created containing a list of active ingredients and excipients and the exact amounts needed of each to prepare the particular prescription. This worksheet should first be double-checked for error and then referred to a checkpoint throughout the preparation of the prescription. As each ingredient is weighed, it should be checked off the worksheet. (This is especially necessary when a formula calls for multiple active ingredients and excipients.) The weights of all active ingredients should be confirmed by the pharmacist or (as individual state law allows) by another pharmacy technician.

There is an extensive list of equipment used in pharmaceutical compounding. When performing any task, you must be able to choose the appropriate tool needed to prepare a quality product. It is important for you as the compounding technician to be familiar with the available tools and their functions.

Equipment and Supplies

Following is a partial list of compounding equipment and their basic functions:

balance—for measuring ingredients

beakers—for measuring ingredients and for mixing or heating ingredients

capsule filling equipment—to prepare capsules

chopper/grinder—to break up solids or ingredients of large particle size

electronic mortar and pestle—for mixing creams and ointments and for reducing particle size

filter paper—to remove particulate matter from a liquid

funnels—to transfer liquids and powders

graduates—for measuring liquids

heat gun—to melt bases and to smooth the tops of troches or suppositories

homogenizer—to reduce particle size and evenly suspend liquids

hotplates—for melting bases

liquid blender—for mixing liquids

magnetic stir plate—for continuous stirring

magnetic stirrers—for continuous stirring

molds—to make troches and suppositories

mortars and pestles—to mix powders and to reduce particle size

    glass—for liquids

    Wedgwood—for powders of significant particle size

    porcelain—for powders

ointment tile—for making creams and ointments

powder blender—to mix powders

refrigerator—for storage ingredients and prescriptions that need cold temperatures

safety glasses—to protect the preparer's eyes from debris

sieves in various mesh sizes—to reduce particle size

spatulas—use for mixing creams and ointments and for retrieving chemicals from the bottle

spray bottles—to dispense cleaning solutions or distilled water

stirring rods—to stir liquids by hand

strainers—to remove particulate from a liquid

thermometers—to control temperature

tongs—to pick up items that should not be handled

tube crimper—to seal ointment tubes

tubes—to dispense creams and ointments

wash bottles—for washing

weigh boats/papers—to weigh ingredients on a balance

weights for calibration—to calibrate a balance

Compounding Facilities

An area suitable for compounding must be established before preparing a compounded prescription. The area should be separate from all other work areas and away from heavy traffic flow. The workspace should be large enough to accommodate all the necessary supplies. It should be clean and free of any clutter. Any object not directly involved in preparing the compound should be removed. All tools and surface areas should be cleaned just prior to use and again when the compound is complete. This can be accomplished by wiping everything down with isopropyl alcohol 70 percent or another suitable cleaning solution. This will safeguard the compounded prescription from possible cross-contamination as well as prevent microbial growth within the final product.

When mixing the active ingredient(s) with the excipient(s), the principle of geometric dilution should be practiced. This is to start with the ingredient of the smallest amount and double the portion by adding the additional ingredients in order of quantity. Each addition should result in a "doubled" amount until all the ingredients are mixed in. This process ensures even distribution of the active ingredient throughout the final product.

Determining the most appropriate dosage form will depend not only on the drug that is being compounded, but on the patient as well. The patient is probably the most important factor to consider when deciding which dosage form to prepare for a compounded prescription. Some common dosage forms that can be effectively compounded are capsules, liquids, transdermal gels, creams, ointments, suppositories, and chewables. Each form will require precise instructions for preparing a quality, efficacious product. (See Figure 9-1.)

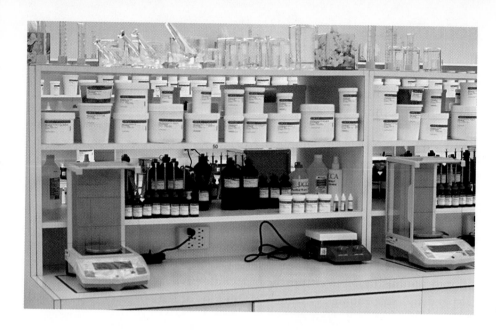

Figure 9-1 The compounding pharmacy

Dosage Forms and Basic Guidelines

There are many types of dosage forms. They include capsules, liquids, solutions, suspensions, emulsions, ointments, suppositories, creams, transdermal gels, and otic and nasal preparations. A discussion of each follows.

CAPSULES

Capsules, as an oral dosage form, have been used for more than a century. The capsule has an important role in drug delivery in that it is extremely versatile and offers a broad range of dosage options for patients. The capsule offers flexibility in dosing to the prescriber as well as to the patient with specific needs.

Capsules can be prepared either by hand or by using a capsule machine. Which method is used will depend on the quantity needed and the physical characteristics of the powders included in the formula.

Using a capsule machine saves time and produces a number of capsules at a time, depending on the size of the machine and the desired quantity. Simply blocking off some of the holes can make a smaller number of capsules.

LIQUIDS

A liquid will be either in the form of a solution or a suspension. A solution is a liquid containing one or more active ingredients that are completely dissolved. A suspension is a liquid containing one or more active ingredients that remain solid and are dispersed evenly throughout the liquid upon being shaken. Solubility is usually the determining factor in the decision of which type of liquid to make.

SOLUTIONS

In an aqueous solution, the water-soluble chemical is dissolved in the water phase of the compound. This may consist of just enough distilled or preserved water to dissolve the drug, or the water may be as much as 50 percent of the final volume. After the drug is completely dissolved in the water, adding flavoring agents and bringing it to the final volume with a sweetening agent such as Ora-Sweet, Simple Syrup, or Karo Syrup may complete the compound. Although the drug is in solution, it may be necessary to shake the liquid before use in order to evenly distribute the flavor.

SUSPENSIONS

A suspension is a liquid preparation that contains insoluble solid particles uniformly dispersed throughout the vehicle. A suspension needs to be shaken prior to administration to ensure the proper dose is dispensed. If a drug is to be suspended, a suspending agent such as Ora-Plus or Karo Syrup will be needed.

EMULSIONS

An emulsion is another type of liquid or semi-solid preparation that can be taken orally or applied topically. Emulsions are prepared whenever two immiscible liquids must be dispensed in the same preparation. An emulsifying agent is used to hold the two together. One part is oil and the other part is aqueous. Emulsions are either water in oil (w/o) or oil in water (o/w), depending on the external phase of the final product. Generally, emulsions that are to be used internally are of the o/w type, whereas emulsions for topical use can be of either type.

Emulsions should be shaken well before use in order to temporarily suspend the aqueous phase into the oil phase and equally distribute the active ingredient(s).

OINTMENTS

An ointment is a semisolid preparation that is usually applied to the skin or to mucosal tissue. An ointment does not penetrate into the skin, but rather stays on top of the skin. Ointments should be soft and easily spread. They should also be smooth in texture, not gritty. Common ointment bases used in compounding include white petrolatum, hydrophilic petrolatum, Aquaphor, hydrous Lanolin, and PEG ointments.

To ensure a smooth ointment, the particle size of a powder being incorporated into the base should be reduced to an impalpable form by comminuting. This can be achieved by using a Wedgwood or porcelain mortar and pestle or by forcing the powder(s) through a size 100 mesh sieve. Once the particle size is reduced, the powder can then be mixed into the base, using geometric dilution. At times it will be necessary to "wet" the powder with a solvent such as glycerin, ethoxydiglycol, or propylene glycol before incorporating them into the base. Other times the drug will be dissolved in oil, such as mineral oil, prior to mixing with the base.

CREAMS

A cream is a soft solid that is opaque and usually applied externally. Creams dissipate into the skin, healing the affected area from the inner layers of the dermis.

Medications are usually suspended or dissolved in a water-soluble base when compounding a cream. A cream must be smooth, and the active ingredients should be dissolved completely in order for them to be totally absorbed into the skin. Cream bases that are available for compounding include vanishing cream base and HRT base, as well as some commercially prepared creams such as Cetaphil, Eucerin, and Lubriderm.

When adding active ingredients to creams, it is critical to practice the principles of geometric dilution to ensure even dispersion. A wetting agent may be necessary; and, again, the volume required to wet the powder should be calculated into the formula when determining the amount of base needed to bring the product to the final desired quantity.

SUPPOSITORIES

A suppository is a solid dosage form that is inserted into the rectum or vagina. The suppository melts and softens or dissolves at body temperature, thus allowing absorption of the medication into the surrounding tissues. Suppositories can either have a systemic effect or a local effect depending on the desired effect expected by the prescriber or on the drug being used. Suppositories can be made in several different shapes and sizes, depending on the patient and the disease state being treated.

When determining which base is most appropriate to use in compounding suppositories, you will have to consider the physical characteristics of the drug ordered as well as the patient. Some of the common bases used for preparing suppositories include fattibase, polybase, and cocoa butter. A drug may either be dissolved in the base or it may need to be suspended, depending on the physical characteristics of the drug being ordered. Whether the drug is dissolved or suspended, the active ingredients and excipients should be added in geometric proportion to ensure that the active ingredient is equally dispersed throughout.

TRANSDERMAL GELS

The transdermal gel is a unique, semisolid dosage form that is becoming increasingly popular. Transdermal gels have special absorption enhancers that "push" the medication through the layers of the skin so that the medication can be absorbed into the bloodstream. The transdermal gel is an especially desirable alternative for pediatric patients, animals that are difficult to "pill" or otherwise medicate, the elderly, and patients who are physically or mentally disabled.

The most common form of compounded transdermal gel therapy is a two-phase vehicle made from pluronic lecithin organogel. It consists of both an oil phase and an aqueous phase, making it a suitable choice for many chemicals. The oil phase, which is lecithin isopropyl palmitate, is generally in a concentration of 22 percent, and the balance is made of poloxamer. Oil soluble drugs should be dissolved in the oil phase, whereas water-soluble drugs should be dissolved in the aqueous phase. The determined amount of drug is dissolved in the appropriate phase, and then the two components are mixed together by using a shearing action. This shear force is necessary for proper micelle formation in the gel. The poloxamer gel is a liquid, which is stored in the refrigerator. When brought to room temperature, it will form a gel. It is important for the final product to be stored at room temperature. Auxiliary labels to this effect (as well as other instructions for the patient, not included on the prescription label) should be placed on the package prior to dispensing.

OTIC

Preparations for the ear are either in a liquid, a powder, or an ointment. Solutions and suspensions are instilled into the ear, whereas ointments are applied to the external ear. Powders are used infrequently, but would usually be administered to the ear canal by a physician. Otic preparations are generally used to treat local infections and the pain associated with them. Other otic products are used to dissolve or remove blockages that can lead to infection.

The vehicles most often used when compounding otic liquids are propylene glycol, glycerin, polyethylene glycol, vegetable oil (especially olive oil), and, occasionally, mineral oil. It is necessary to use a viscous liquid such as one of these, since it will adhere to the ear canal. Water and alcohol may be used as a vehicle, but are typically used as solvents for the drugs being compounded or used in an irrigating solution. The physical characteristics of the ingredients used in compounding otic preparations that need to be considered include solubility, viscosity, and tonicity. Almost always, a preservative will be used when preparing an otic preparation. Although otic preparations need not be sterile, it is important for the pharmacy technician to follow quality control procedures for preventing cross contamination or microbial growth in the compound. Many chemicals used in otic preparations are soluble in the vehicles used in compounding them. Due to the general viscosity of these products, a suspending agent is usually not necessary if the drug is insoluble.

When compounding a liquid for otic use, the drug and any preservatives or other excipients are accurately weighed and then dissolved or mixed with approximately three-quarters of the vehicle. When the drug is completely dissolved or evenly suspended, the preparation is then brought to final volume with more of the vehicle. When an ointment is being prepared, the drug and any other ingredients are accurately weighed and then mixed into the base by using the principles of geometric dilution.

NASAL

Preparations for nasal administration are in the form of solutions, suspensions, gels, or ointments. These preparations may be used locally or systemically, depending on the nature of the drug and the vehicle it is in.

In addition to the active ingredient, several excipients will most likely be used. These include the vehicle, buffers, preservatives, and tonicity-adjusting agents. Since nasal preparations are generally dispensed in multiuse containers,

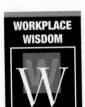

WORKPLACE WISDOM

This chapter is just an overview of the specialty practice of compounding in community pharmacy. Specific techniques have not been included, as they are too advanced and detailed for the scope of this book. For an in-depth look at extemporaneous compounding and step-by-step procedures, please review *Compounding for Technicians*, published by Prentice Hall Health.

it is necessary to use a preservative. The pH must be adjusted so that maximum stability is obtained. Two common vehicles used for nasal solutions are sodium chloride 0.9 percent and sterile water for injection.

Ingredients for nasal preparations should be sterile, and aseptic technique should be used to make them. Sterility may be obtained by filtration or autoclaving. If a drug is water soluble, it will be dissolved in a portion of the vehicle and the liquid will be brought to final volume with the vehicle. A suspension will require that the active ingredient and any excipients be mixed by using geometric dilution with a suspending agent and then brought to final volume with the appropriate vehicle. Mixing the active ingredient and any excipients with the base by using the principles of geometric dilution makes nasal gels or ointments.

Quality control procedures should be observed when making nasal preparations. Prior to dispensing, the pharmacist should determine clarity, pH, and correct volume or weight.

VETERINARY COMPOUNDING

Veterinary compounding is one of the fastest growing areas of pharmaceutical compounding. Medication doses are usually calculated on the basis of milligrams per kilogram. Because of the vast difference in the size and physiology of animals, this makes appropriate dosing nearly impossible when using manufactured products.

The same principles used in human compounding of medications apply to veterinary compounding. Stability, solubility, drug availability, dosage form choices, cost effectiveness of drug sources, and quality of final product are all factors to be considered before attempting to compound for animals.

In addition to capsules, flavored liquids, transdermal gels, and suppositories, the chewable treat is another dosage form available for pharmaceutical compounding. A chewable form made from a base of ground food product and gelatin mixed with the active ingredient is an excellent choice for animals. Some flavor choices for these chewable forms include liver, tuna, salmon, shrimp, chicken, and beef. Again, solubility is taken into consideration when preparing the treat form. If a drug is water-soluble it can be incorporated into the gelatin phase of the compound. If insoluble it will be mixed in geometric proportion with the solid, or food, phase of the compound and then mixed with the gelatin. The mixture is then forced by way of a syringe or other means into precalibrated molds. The final product is a soft chewable form that can be offered to the animal as a treat, or mixed in with a small amount of the animal's favorite food, for consumption.

CONCLUSION

Extemporaneous compounding is a special service provided by a number of community-based pharmacies. Additional training, skills, and practice are required for a pharmacy technician to assist in compounding, but compounding also provides a number of advanced professional opportunities for those who pursue these skills.

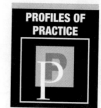

CHAPTER REVIEW QUESTIONS

1. What are some of the factors that must be considered before compounding a prescription medication?

    a. cost effectiveness, availability, solubility, and stability

    b. suspending agent, profit margin, and ease of preparation

    c. proper tools, adequate support personnel, and time

    d. insurance reimbursement, available flavoring agents, active ingredient, and source

2. The extemporaneous compounding of prescription medications differs from traditional pharmacy in that it involves a relationship between:

    a. mother, father, and child

    b. patient, practitioner, and pharmacist

    c. pharmacist, patient, and insurance carrier

    d. doctor, nurse, and patient

3. Pharmacy is the only profession that allows the extemporaneous compounding of chemicals for:

    a. resale

    b. veterinarians

    c. therapeutic care

    d. use in physician's offices

4. Of the following reference materials, which would not be necessary in a compounding facility?

    a. *Remington's Pharmaceutical Sciences*

    b. *The Merck Manual*

    c. *Drug Facts and Comparisons*

    d. *Pharmacy Times Magazine*

5. Which area of the compounding procedure has the greatest potential for error?

    a. pharmaceutical calculations

    b. retrieving the proper chemical

    c. selecting the proper vehicle

    d. choosing the best flavor

6. Who is responsible for checking the calculations performed for a specific formula?

    a. another technician

    b. the pharmacist

    c. the person who performs the calculations

    d. ancillary personnel

7. The compilation of ingredients and instructions is known as the:

    a. worksheet

    b. menu

    c. formula

    d. list

8. In order to avoid cross-contamination, the compounding area should be cleaned:

    a. before the procedure

    b. after the procedure

    c. daily

    d. both before and after the procedure

9. Transdermal gels in the form of a pluronic lecithin organogel are considered to be:

    a. an emulsion

    b. an ointment

    c. a cream

    d. a suspension

10. Which of the following types of mortar and pestle would be the ideal choice when working with liquids?

    a. porcelain

    b. glass

    c. Wedgwood

    d. any of the above

Resources and References

1. Allen, Loyd V. Jr., Ph.D. *The Art, Science, and Technology of Pharmaceutical Compounding.* Washington, DC: American Pharmaceutical Association, 1998.

2. Hoover, John E., Ed. *Remington's Pharmaceutical Sciences*, 15th Edition.

3. *Pharmaceutical Necessities.* Easton, PA: Mack Publishing Company, 1975.

4. Allen, Loyd V. Jr., Ph.D. "A History of Pharmaceutical Compounding," *Secundum Artem*, Volume 1, Number 1. Minneapolis, MN: Paddock Laboratories.

5. Allen, Loyd V. Jr., Ph.D. "Pharmaceutical Compounding Calculations." *Secundum Artem*, Volume 5, Number 2. Minneapolis, MN: Paddock Laboratories.

6. Allen, Loyd V. Jr., Ph.D. "Pharmacy Compounding Equipment," *Secundum Artem*, Volume 4, Number 3. Minneapolis, MN: Paddock Laboratories.

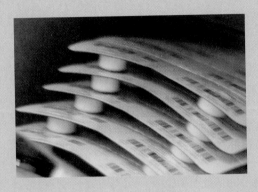

Institutional Pharmacy Operations

L earning Objectives

After completing this chapter, you should be able to:

- Describe the institutional pharmacy practice setting.
- Define the tasks that pharmacy technicians perform in institutional settings.
- Describe the advantages of a unit dose system.
- List the necessary components of a medication order.
- Compare the duties of a technician with those of a pharmacist in accepting a medication order in an institutional setting.
- Compare a centralized and a decentralized unit dose system.
- List the benefits of automated dosing systems.
- Describe the duties of a technician and those of a pharmacist in filling a medication order in an institutional setting.

INTRODUCTION

Institutional pharmacy describes the range of services provided to residents of nursing homes, hospitals, hospice, and other long-term care facilities. Within an institutional setting, the pharmacist takes responsibility for the patients' medication related needs and ensures that the patients' medications are appropriate, effective, safe, and used correctly. The institutional pharmacist also identifies, resolves, and prevents medication related problems. The pharmacy technician working in an institution must be keenly aware of institutional policies and procedures as well as state and federal law. Because working with less supervision is common in most institutional settings, the professional technician must also be familiar with dosing, compounding, IV administration, and other drug related procedures.

Institutional Pharmacy

The institutional pharmacy provides around-the-clock delivery service. It also provides prescription drugs in individually packaged blister packs (unit dose packages) so that they are dispensed in an easy and safe manner. Many institutional pharmacists constantly check patients' drug interactions to avoid possible duplications of treatment and adverse reactions. This makes the institutional pharmacy a principal defense against medical errors and helps give the patient quality care. An institutional setting is a setting in which the patient stays at the pharmacy location and can be more closely monitored for special care.

Institutional pharmacists not only counsel patients; they also provide information and recommendations to doctors and other caregivers, review patients' drug regimens, and oversee medication distribution services.

Institutional pharmacists may work with nurses, physical therapists, dietitians, physicians, and other caregivers to discuss the drug therapy of patients and to prevent and solve problems. Working with caregivers is required by federal law in many settings. Several studies have been done showing that, in most cases, the physician heeds the counsel of the pharmacist on drug therapy recommendations.

Institutional pharmacy teams are committed to providing products and services 24 hours a day, 365 days a year. Institutional pharmacies address emergency as well as regular needs. They have designed special practices with protocols that enable them to provide medication within two hours.

Institutional pharmacists and technicians use controlled dispensing systems to ensure that patients have the right drugs at the right time and in the proper dosage and form. These systems enable the staff to administer medications with ease and in proper pre-measured doses. This enhances compliance, saves time, helps prevent medication errors, and makes it possible to track medication usage. Medication carts, filled and delivered by technicians, enable the patients to get the right medication at the right time.

Institutional pharmacies allow unused, unopened products to be returned for credit (where permitted by state). With the return of unused, unopened drugs, a patient's medication changes do not result in unused products going to waste. This is a very cost-effective practice.

Institutional pharmacy services are comprehensive in scope and intensity. Elderly, seriously ill, or chronically ill patients who are often frail and have multiple chronic conditions need more attention than healthier, ambulatory patients suffering from just one condition. As an institutionalized patient's condition constantly changes, the frequent updating of drug regimens is required. (See Figure 10-1.)

LONG-TERM CARE FACILITIES

The federal government has recognized the distinctive feature of the long-term care pharmacy, passed laws to protect the health and well-being of institutional residents (OBRA 1987, OBRA 1990), and put rules in place (HCFA'S 1990 nursing home regulations). These rules have ascertained that

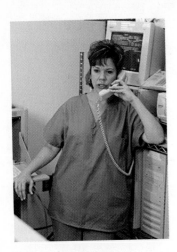

Figure 10-1 The institutional pharmacy technician

drug therapy services for institutional patients are best delivered by the long-term care pharmacist.

Long-term care pharmacists perform thorough drug therapy review, since they have access to comprehensive information about the patients. Each patient's drug therapy is reviewed monthly to make sure that the therapy is appropriate to the patient's diagnoses, change in condition, and goals for treatment. Federal law requires the pharmacist to perform a monthly drug review (DRR) on each patient. The pharmacists look for drug–drug interactions, drug–disease interactions, and drug–food interactions. This is made possible because of the pharmacist's access to the patient's complete medical record, including diagnosis, doctors' orders, lab results, treatment records, and other important information. This information also helps the pharmacist when he meets the patient. When meeting the patient, the pharmacist may assess the patient face-to-face to see if medications are causing any side effects or health problems.

Job Responsibilities

In order to allow pharmacists to focus on the medication-related problems of their patients and to provide the best pharmaceutical care, many tasks in the institutional care facility that were once performed by the pharmacist are now delegated to qualified support staff, including pharmacy technicians. The pharmacy technician, under the supervision of the pharmacist, can perform a wide range of tasks. These tasks (where allowed by the laws of the state in which the technician works) may involve a variety of components of the pharmacy practice, including, but not limited to, the following:

1. Data Collection and Reporting
   - Prepare patient satisfaction assessments.
   - Compile continuous quality improvement data.
   - Manage drug inventory.
   - Perform formulary maintenance.
   - Prepare billing statements.
2. Survey and Inspections
   - Conduct medication room inspections.
   - Conduct narcotic audits.
   - Check emergency boxes and replace outdated medications.
   - Check orders for completeness.
   - Inspect and service crash carts.
3. Education
   - Assist in facility meetings.
   - Help organize and maintain the medical library.
   - Provide in-service training and continuing education for facility personnel.

4. Maintenance
   • Assist in the maintenance of devices (fax machine, automated dispensing systems, and so on).
5. Dispensing and Inventory
   • Order medication stock.
   • Package medications.
   • Prepare intravenous solutions.
   • Fill and label prescriptions.

To make sure that technicians are properly trained and their performance is evaluated, the supervising pharmacist will provide a written job description of the functions performed by the pharmacy technicians, according to regulations in the state in which the technician is practicing.

The initial orientation and training for pharmacy technicians should include information about properly performing their assigned functions, the unique needs of institutionalized patients, and relevant regulations.

The pharmacy technician also needs to have ongoing training and education. The technician should be given periodic evaluations of his job performance.

WORKPLACE WISDOM

No task delegated to a pharmacy technician may involve performing a final check of a medication to the patient or any task that requires the professional judgment of a pharmacist.

SPECIAL TERMS

Advisory committee is a medication management committee established to advise the quality assurance committee.

Medication-related error is any preventable medication-related event that adversely affects a patient in a nursing home and that is related to professional practice or health care products, procedures, or systems, including prescribing, prescription order communications, product labeling, packaging and nomenclature, compounding, dispensing distribution, administration, education, monitoring, and use.

Nursing home is an adult care home licensed and governed by the state and subject to federal regulations.

Potential medication-related error is a medication-related error that has not yet adversely affected a patient in the institution, but has the potential to do so if left unnoticed.

Quality assurance (Q & A) committee is established within an institution in accordance with federal and state regulations to identify circumstances requiring quality assessment and quality assurance activities and to develop and implement an appropriate plan of action to correct deficiencies in quality of care.

The practice of pharmacy in an institutional setting is evolving just as fast as, if not faster than, in ambulatory settings. Innovations in medications, drug delivery systems, information systems, and patient care provide technicians opportunities for more training, education, and responsibility in the health care system.

Processing Medication Orders

Institutional pharmacy settings are, basically, pharmacies located in the "home" of the patients served there. This home can be a hospital, nursing home, or hospice. Several differences distinguish the institutional pharmacy practice from the ambulatory. From the writing, receiving, and filling to the dispensing of medications, these differences can be challenges to technicians unless there is adequate training beforehand.

RECEIVING THE ORDER

Just as in an ambulatory setting, no medications are dispensed in an institutional setting without a prescription. In an institution, the prescription (medication order) is not handed to the patient to be filled, but entered into his chart, filled, billed, and delivered to the patient.

The order may arrive in the pharmacy in one of the following ways:

- The pharmacist may be handed the order directly.
- The order may be faxed to the pharmacy.
- Orders for medication may be sent through the institutional computer system.
- A technician may be assigned to collect medication orders from many sources throughout the institution. (See Figure 10-2.)

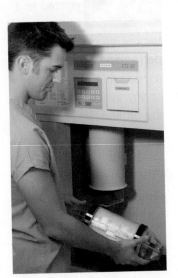

Figure 10-2 Receiving a medication order

ORDER REQUIREMENTS

There are some differences in the requirements of a medication order compared with a prescription, but the reasons are self-evident. (See Figure 10-3.)

Patient Information:
  Name
  Room/bed number
  Hospital ID number
  Birth date/age

Medication Information:
  Name
  Dose
  Frequency of administration
  Route
  Signature of prescriber
  Date and hour the order was written

ORDER VERIFICATION

Technicians practicing in institutional settings may be assigned to collect and accept medication orders and even review the orders for completeness. These orders are called unverified and cannot be processed until they have been verified by a pharmacist.

PHYSICIAN'S ORDER WORKSHEET

NOTE: *Person initiating entry should write legibly, date the form using (Mo./Day/Yr.), enter time, sign, and indicate their title.*

USE BALL POINT PEN (PRESS FIRMLY)

Date	Time	Treatment
		③

	PHYSICIAN'S ORDER WORKSHEET	Distribution: (Original) Medical Record Copy (Plies 3, 2, & 1) Pharmacy	**T-5**

Figure 10-3 Sample medication order

CHOOSING THE MEDICATION

Within an institutional setting, there may be many types of medication distribution systems. This is especially true of a hospital setting, where there may even be multiple pharmacies. Some more common types of medication distribution systems are floor stock, individual, and unit-dose.

FLOOR STOCK

Medications are kept on each floor for patient distribution. This system is prone to errors and diversion. However, in recent times, computers have

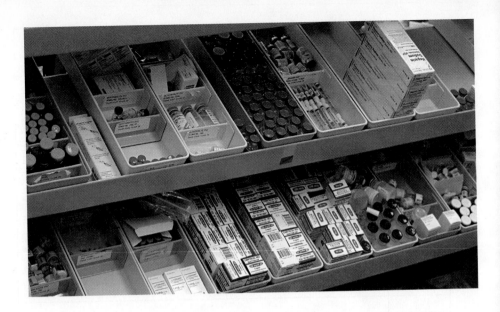

Figure 10-4 Floor stock medicine

made this system much easier to monitor and fill. The technician will stock the floor unit with a predetermined bulk supply after the pharmacist checks the order. The computerized system will track the inventory, monitor who has accessed the unit, and even bill the patient. This system can generate refill orders to the technician, and the process can begin again. (See Figure 10-4.)

INDIVIDUAL

This system is the most inefficient because of waste and is harder to track. After reviewing medication orders for a floor, the technician would take the medications to that floor (after the pharmacist has verified the orders). This would be a several days' supply, and once opened, the medication cannot be returned to the pharmacy.

UNIT-DOSE

This is the most efficient distribution system and makes it very easy to track a patient's medications. Each medication order is filled in the pharmacy in as close to administration form as possible. Not more than a 24-hour supply is dispensed at one time. Scanners may be used to track and bill for the medications when they are dispensed. The unit-dose system centralizes medication preparation into the pharmacy itself, cuts the amount of time the nursing staff spends preparing medications, and greatly reduces waste.

Clearly, a unit-dose system requires more technician involvement. In a centralized pharmacy, technicians may have workstations for unit dose (tablets, capsules, and liquids), IV, sterile, chemo, injections, and compounding. (See Figure 10-5.)

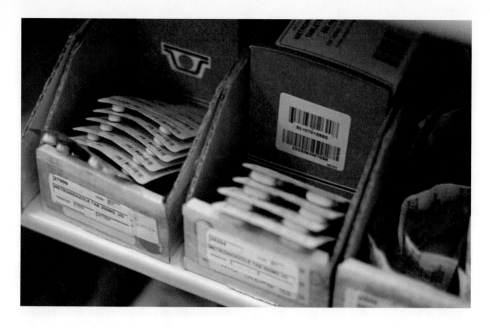

Figure 10-5 Unit-dosed medicine

FINAL CHECK

The final check is the sole domain of the pharmacist. No medications may be dispensed without the pharmacist's final approval. In an institutional setting, this is a relatively simple process. The pharmacist will need the original medication order and the labeled container filled with the prescribed medication. Once the pharmacist gives his approval, the medication may be sent to the proper ward or floor and dispensed to the patient.

Filling Medication Orders

One of the most basic duties of a pharmacy technician in any setting is the filling of prescriptions or medication orders. In the institutional setting, filling is more than counting and basic measuring.

HAND COUNTING

Just as in an ambulatory setting, medications may be counted out in an institutional setting. The same care must be taken to match lot/UPC numbers and expiration dates. The technician performing this task needs to keep the spatula and the counting tray clean at all times. Special care should be taken when counting cytotoxic or chemo-drugs. A good technician will count twice, especially when counting C-II medications.

AUTOMATED COUNTERS

There are many different counting machines, from the fairly simple to the extremely expensive and complicated. Technicians are required to operate and

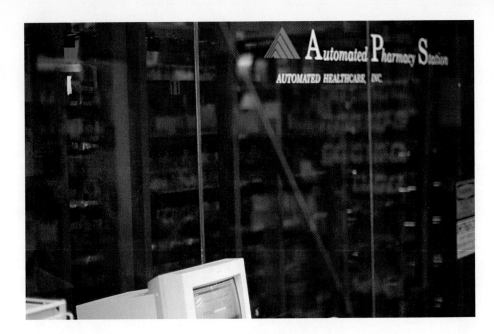

Figure 10-6 Automated counting machine

maintain these systems on a daily basis. These machines are popular because they are efficient, reduce errors, and can also reduce diversion. An important point to remember is that these machines are only as accurate as the technicians operating them. At no time should a technician override a machine's built-in checking system. Close attention must be paid to any policy and procedure pertaining to the operation of automated dispensing equipment.(See Figure 10-6.)

UNIT DOSE SYSTEMS

Unit dose systems can be centralized, decentralized, or a combination. A centralized system is operated out of one pharmacy location. All medications are prepared and dispensed from one location. Technicians can be assigned to prepare IVs, TPNs, injectables, compounding, or repackaging. They will operate different dispensing equipment. Just like in an ambulatory setting, the right medication must get to the right patient. The dosage forms are more varied, and the dose size is individualized.

The decentralized system operates out of more than one, and perhaps even several different locations, each responsible for a section of the institution. This system may be necessary in some institutions with larger populations. The down side to this system is the duplication of staff, inventory, and equipment.

UNIT DOSE PACKAGING

Pharmacy technicians are charged with maintaining the unit dose systems in an institution. This requires selecting medications and preparing them for dispensing, similar to an ambulatory setting, but with an added step.

Medication carts are filled with the medications for each patient in their individual drawer. Since many medications do not come in unit-dose form, it is the pharmacy technician's responsibility to prepare all medications. The goal is to prepare each medication as close to its dispensing form as possible. These doses are not labeled for a particular patient, but must be clearly labeled as to strength and name. As with any repackaging, strict attention to detail must be observed. Each dose must be identifiable up to the time it is administered. All medications must remain sanitary, and in some cases (such as IV or injections), sterile.

Some medications cannot be unit dosed. These would include drops, ointments, and creams. In these cases, the medications must be labeled for the individual patients. The label will contain the following information:

- patient's name
- location (floor, room, and bed numbers)
- drug (name and strength)
- date

BAR-CODING

The Food and Drug Administration (FDA) has established a rule that bar-coding is mandatory on medications. This rule applies to all prescription drug products, including biological products, vaccines (except for physician samples), and OTC drugs that are commonly used and dispensed in a hospital. Standardized bar codes would also be required on prescription drug products used in other settings, such as retail pharmacies.

With the continuous growth of automation and increase in drugs, the FDA deemed it necessary to create a method of reducing medication problems through using state-of-the-art technology to reduce the number of medication errors in hospitals and other health care settings. Bar-coding and scanning addresses the "five rights" related to patient safety in preventing medication errors: the right medication, right dose, right patient, right time, and right route.

The required bar code contains the National Drug Code (NDC) number and unique, identifying information about the drug that is to be dispensed to the patient, in a linear bar code, as part of the drug label. The code allows for the further addition of even more information as technology progresses.

IV, TPN, AND INJECTABLES

Technicians filling orders for IV medications or TPNs need specialized training. There is a plethora of machines and measuring systems available; but, again, the equipment is only as good as the operator. Technicians filling these kinds of medications work with less supervision, do a lot more calculating, and therefore have to be well trained. There are several accreditations and certifications available for technicians choosing to specialize in this area, and technicians wishing to perform this type of work should take advantage of those opportunities. (See Figure 10-7.)

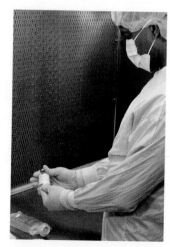

Figure 10-7 Preparation of sterile products

Patient Care

Modern patient care requires the exchange of a large amount of information. Until recently, pharmacy technicians were silent, behind-the-scene workers. Patient care, to them, was patient billing and cash register tending. As the practice of pharmacy evolved, so did the role of the pharmacy technician. Pharmacy technicians manage a great deal of patient information themselves. The technician can be a valuable resource to the other members of the patient's health care team if he learns how to communicate essential information effectively.

In an institutional setting, technicians have less contact with the patients, but their roles are still integral to each patient's health. There are many more opportunities in an institutional setting than in most ambulatory settings for a technician to play an active part in the improvement of patient care. Some institutional pharmacies allow technicians on their formulary committees. Others use technicians to gather and evaluate patient statistics. The opportunities are growing as the pharmacy industry grows. Technicians should actively participate in the administration of the pharmacy where they work as much as they can. The more useful the technician becomes to other members of the health care team, the better will be the patient care they are providing. Freeing up more of the pharmacist's time, which enables him to spend that time on patient counseling and other health care collaborations, is also a great way for technicians to provide patient care.

Teamwork

No doubt you've heard the phrase "It takes a village to raise a child." You can also say that it takes a team to improve a patient's health. If a pharmacy is to run efficiently, everyone on the team has to work together. Professional technicians know how to leave their egos at the door. After all, technicians are support staff. On a good team, everyone knows their job and their place. Understanding the team concept can also help avoid personality conflicts and petty issues. With everyone focused on the patient and working to keep the pharmacy running smoothly, the patient will receive the best care possible.

Every team needs a captain, and in a pharmacy setting the pharmacist assumes that position. Technicians must always remember that no moves are made without the captain calling the play. All medication orders must be reviewed by a pharmacist before the dispensing process can begin. A technician's work should be evaluated often by a pharmacist. Good communication on both sides allows for constructive criticism and opens the door for positive suggestions. It also allows for the safe transmission of information that might be critical to a patient's health.

Communication Tips

- Know whom you are talking to. Know as much as you can about the person you are addressing. After working with a person for awhile, this becomes easier. If you want them to "hear" you, you may need to adjust your choice of words to those that are on their level of thinking.

- Be clear and precise. Pharmacy is a fast-paced, time-sensitive practice. Don't beat around the bush. Know what you intend to say before you say it. Respect other people's time. When imparting technical information, clarity and precision are of the utmost importance.

- Avoid personalizing a problem. If a problem is only a problem for you, then it is your problem. If the situation you see as a problem negatively affects the patients or other people in the pharmacy, then you need to act. In teamwork, the individual takes a back seat to the needs of the team. With the team focused on the patient, this is a win-win situation.

- Listen. After you have said what you came to say, listen to the response. There might be information there that will help you. Listening is the difference between having a conversation and talking "at" someone.

- Be honest and fair. Whether it is a mistake or a success, tell it like it is. Mistakes cannot be corrected or avoided in the future if they are not acknowledged in the present. When there is praise to be handed out, share as much as you honestly can with your associates. No one person on a team wins; the whole team wins, or the whole team loses. Honesty, especially when dealing with errors, can lead to solutions, improvements, and healings.

Pharmacy practice has become much too involved not to require teamwork. Patient care has become much too complicated to be handled by prescribers alone. As a collaborative effort, a health care team, working closely together in a professional manner, can make significant improvements in a patients' overall health and well being.

CONCLUSION

Although filling prescriptions and medication orders is basically the same task, institutional pharmacy practice is more varied than community pharmacy practice. Technicians will be working with several distribution systems and not just repackaging medications for specific patients, but also bulk repackaging for floors and patient care areas. Institutional technicians deal in sterile and aseptic techniques, cytotoxins and chemo drugs, as well as a variety of automatic dispensing systems.

PROFILES
OF PRACTICE

C an you decipher these sample medication orders? (See Figures 10-8 and 10-9.)

16285 CH-7239 (FEB. 03)	

PHYSICIAN'S ORDER WORKSHEET

NOTE: *Person initiating entry should write legibly, date the form using (Mo./Day/Yr.), enter time, sign, and indicate their title.*

USE BALL POINT PEN (PRESS FIRMLY)

77004513   314 B
McGraw, Phillip A.
4/20/60
Dr. A. H. Kline

Date	Time	Treatment
12/4	14:45	1) Metoprolol 25mg po bid
		2) Prednisone 20mg po bid
		Dr. AHKline
		x1444
		③

	PHYSICIAN'S ORDER WORKSHEET	Distribution: (Original) Medical Record Copy (Plies 3, 2, & 1) Pharmacy	**T-5**

Figure 10-8   Sample medication order

		16285

PHYSICIAN'S ORDER WORKSHEET

NOTE: *Person initiating entry should write legibly, date the form using (Mo./Day/Yr.), enter time, sign, and indicate their title.*

USE BALL POINT PEN (PRESS FIRMLY)

16285
CH-7239
(FEB. 03)

01456830   204 A
Marshall, Peter F.
10/18/48
Dr. P. Patel

Date	Time	Treatment
3/12	⏰	Norvasc 5mg po QD
		P. Patel ⌀ 3145
		③

	PHYSICIAN'S ORDER WORKSHEET	Distribution: (Original) Medical Record Copy (Plies 3, 2, & 1) Pharmacy	T-5

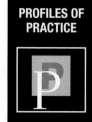

PROFILES OF PRACTICE

Figure 10-9 Sample medication order

CHAPTER REVIEW QUESTIONS

1. Long-term care pharmacists perform a drug therapy review for each patient; how often is this done?

   a. weekly
   b. monthly
   c. semimonthly
   d. quarterly

2. Which of the following was passed by the federal government to protect the health and well being of institutional residents?

   a. OBRA 1987
   b. FEDA 1981
   c. NOVA 1956
   d. OBRA 1945

3. An adult care home that is licensed and governed by state and federal regulations is what?

   a. nursing home
   b. adult day care
   c. homeless shelter
   d. senior center

4. A medication management committee established to advise the quality assurance committee is called:

   a. safe drug committee
   b. pharmacy technician committee
   c. advisory committee
   d. pharmacist committee

5. Once a medication order is packaged in a unit-dose container, it must be:

   a. rushed to the patient
   b. taken to the attending nurse
   c. properly stored until called for
   d. checked by a pharmacist before being dispensed

6. Pharmacy technicians may collect medication orders from:

   a. fax machines
   b. the institutional computer system
   c. prescribers throughout the institution
   d. all of the above

7. The most efficient medication delivery system in an institutional pharmacy is:

   a. individual
   b. floor-stock
   c. unit dose
   d. bulk

8. The benefit of an automated dispensing system is that it:

   a. is cost effective
   b. reduces errors when operated properly
   c. helps reduce diversion
   d. all of the above

9. In an institutional setting, a technician may do all the following, except:

   a. operate automated dispensing machines
   b. repackage medications for unit dosing
   c. fill medication carts
   d. give the OK for medications to leave the pharmacy

10. Which medication cannot be repackaged as a unit dose?

   a. C-II medications
   b. liquid medications
   c. eye drops
   d. reconstituted powders

Resources and References

1. Reifman, Noah. *Certification Review for Pharmacy Technicians, 6th Ed.* Evergreen, CO: Ark Pharmaceutical Consultants, Inc., 2002.

2. American Pharmacist Association. *Pharmacy Technician Workbook and Certification Review.* Englewood, CO: Morton Publishing, 2001.

3. American Society of Health System Pharmacists. *Manual for Pharmacy Technicians.* Bethesda, MD: ASHP, 1998.

4. American Society of Health System Pharmacists. *Pharmacy Technician Certification Review and Exam.* Bethesda, MD: ASHP, 1998.

5. Ballington, Don. *Pharmacy Practice.* St. Paul, MN: EMC Paradigm, 1999.

6. Ballington, Don. *Pharmacy Practice for Technicians.* St. Paul, MN: EMC Paradigm, 2003.

7. Cowen, D. and W. Helfand. *Pharmacy: An Illustrated History.* New York: Harry N. Abrams, Incorporated, 1990.

8. Lambert, Anita. *Advanced Pharmacy Practice for Technicians.* Clifton Park, NY: Delmar, 2002.

9. Ansel, H.C. *Introduction to Pharmaceutical Dosage Forms.* Philadelphia, PA: Lea & Febiger, 1995.

10. The American Medical Association. *Know Your Drugs and Medications.* New York: The Reader's Digest Association, 1991.

11. Facts and Comparisons. "Homepage." 04 January 2004. *http://www.factsandcomparisons.com*

12. Food and Drug Administration. "Homepage." 04 January 2004. *http://www.fda.gov*

Institutional Pharmacy Calculations

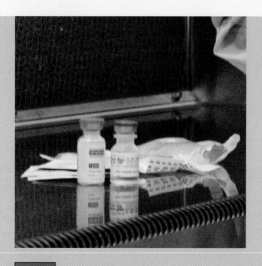

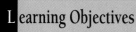
Learning Objectives

After completing this chapter, you should be able to:

- Show calculations commonly used in an institutional setting.
- Calculate the quantity of active ingredient needed for each preparation.
- Determine the rate of flow for IV meds.
- Calculate the volume of electrolytes to add to a TPN.
- Discuss and calculate dilution technique.

INTRODUCTION

Being able to calculate mathematical equations in an institutional practice setting such as the IV room is an essential skill. All proficient technicians have excellent math skills. In the following pages are some examples of math problems with their solutions that you may encounter while working in an institutional pharmacy. These skills will also come handy in many other aspects of pharmacy.

Note: This chapter does not cover basic math principles. For a more in-depth review, refer to Pharmacy Calculations in the Pharmacy Technician Series, published by Prentice Hall Health.

Calculating gtts/min

Drops/minute is primarily a nursing function. Pharmacy usually uses ml/hour or ml/min. However, the IV technician should be able to perform this type of calculation.

Formula A:

$$\frac{\text{total volume}}{\text{total time (min)}} \times \text{drop factor} = \text{gtts/min}$$

EXAMPLE 11.1   A 250 ml Nipride drip is to be infused over 60 minutes. The IV set has a drop factor of 5 gtts/ml. How many drops per minutes should the patient receive? Look at the given information. The given information in the problem is as follows:

- the amount to be infused
- the time to be infused
- drop factor

Use formula A and plug in the given information:

$$\frac{\text{total volume}}{\text{total time (min)}} \times \text{drop factor} = \text{gtts/min}$$

$$\frac{250 \text{ ml}}{60 \text{ min}} \times \frac{5 \text{ gtts}}{1 \text{ ml}} = \text{gtts/min}$$ (Did you notice that the mls cancel out giving you gtts/min?)

20.83 gtts/min ← *answer*

IV Flow Rates

This is useful in determining how many IV bags that a patient will need in a 24-hour period.

The following formula can be adapted for a couple of occasions:

- when an entire bag is being infused
- how many mls are infused after a set time

$$\text{Rate} \frac{\text{(ml)}}{\text{(hr)}} = \frac{\text{amount to be infused (ml)}}{\text{time to be infused (hr)}}$$

EXAMPLE 11.2   An IV has a flow rate of 50 ml/hour. How long will a 1-liter IV bag last? How many bags will the patient need in a 24-hour period?

1. Convert the 1-liter bag to milliliters (mls):

$$1 \text{ liter} = 1000 \text{ ml}$$

Set up the proportion:

$$\frac{50 \text{ ml}}{1 \text{ hr}} = \frac{1000 \text{ ml}}{x \text{ hr}}$$ Cross multiply and solve for *x*.

$$1000 = 50 x$$

$$x = 20 \text{ hours}$$

Therefore, the patient will need two (2) IV bags to get them through a 24-hour period.

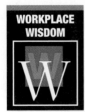

WORKPLACE WISDOM

Make sure that the labels are matched up together on the top and together on the bottom when solving flow rates. Also, always assume 60 gtts = 1 ml, unless noted otherwise on the order.

Use the following formula when a concentration is given:

$$\frac{\text{desired dosage (want)}}{\text{dosage available (have)}} = \frac{\text{rate (mg)}}{\text{(ml)}}$$

EXAMPLE 11.3 A physician wants to infuse a 1-liter NS bag that contains 10-gram Oxacillin at a rate of 400 mg/hr. What is the rate of the bag? How long will the IV bag last? Convert 10 grams of Oxacillin to x mg of Oxacillin.

$$\frac{1 \text{ gram}}{1000 \text{ mg}} = \frac{10 \text{ grams}}{x \text{ mg}}$$

$$x = 10000 \text{ mg of Oxacillin}$$

Determine concentration per ml:

$$\frac{10000 \text{ mg of Oxacillin}}{1000 \text{ ml NS}} = 10 \text{ mg/ml}$$

Set up the equation using the following formula:

$$\frac{400 \text{ mg/hr}}{10 \text{ mg/ml}} = x$$

$$400 \div 10 = 40 \text{ ml/hr (rate)}$$

How long will an IV bag last?

$$1000 \text{ ml} \div 40 \text{ mg/hr} = 25 \text{ hours}$$

Milliequivalents/TPNs

Most students panic when asked to calculate a TPN. But in reality, if you take your time and work through the problem in a methodical way, it's nothing more than a couple of alligations and a couple of ratio/proportions (see Table 11-1).

EXAMPLE 11.4 Name: Baby Smith   Weight: 1 KG
A physician writes an order for a TPN to be infused at a rate of 3.3 ml/hr over a 24-hour period.

TABLE 11-1   The TPN Order

Components	Amount Required	Amount to be added (mls)
Amino Acid (Trophamine 6%)	2.5 gm	1. _____
Dextrose 70%	12.5%	2. _____
Sodium Chloride	6 meq	3. _____
Potassium Phosphate	2.8 meq	4. _____
Potassium Chloride	2 meq	5. _____
Magnesium Sulfate	3 meq	6. _____
Calcium Gluconate	3.2 meq	7. _____
Pediatric MVI	6.5 ml	8. _____
Trace Elements	0.1 ml	9. _____
Heparin	0.5 unit/ml of TAV	10. _____
SWFI	_____	11. _____
TAV (Total Actual Volume)		12. _____

The following supplies are available in the pharmacy:

Trophamine 6%

Dextrose 70%

Sterile Water

Lipids 20%

Sodium Chloride	4 meq/ml
Sodium Acetate	2 meq/ml
Sodium Phosphate	4 meq/ml
Potassium Phosphate	4.4 meq/ml
Potassium Chloride	2 meq/ml
Potassium Acetate	2 meq/ml
Magnesium Sulfate	4.06 meq/ml
Calcium Gluconate	0.47 meq/ml
Heparin	100 units/ml

This looks a lot more difficult than it really is. Let's break it down systematically.

- We need the TAV (total actual volume) before we can start the problem.
  The rate is 3.3 and the TPN is run over 24 hours.
  TAV = 3.3 × 24 = 79.2 ml ← answer to #12

Let's figure out how much Aminosyn is needed. We want 2.5 grams of trophamine. Trophamine comes as a 6% solution. We have all the information that we need. Six percent means that it is 6 grams in 100 ml.
Set this problem up as a ratio/proportion:

$$\frac{6 \text{ grams}}{100 \text{ ml}} = \frac{2.5 \text{ grams}}{x \text{ ml}}$$

Solve for x:

$$250 = 6x$$
$$x = 41.67 \text{ ml} \leftarrow \text{answer to #1}$$

- Now for the Dextrose. This is an alligation. We are diluting a percent strength solution to a different percentage. Our stock solution is Dextrose 70%. Our diluent is SWFI (Dextrose 0%).

70%		12.5% − 0% = 12.5 12.5 parts of Dextrose 70%
	12.5%	
0%		70% − 12.5% = 57.5 57.5 parts of Water

12.5 + 57.5 = 70 parts total

Then set this up as a ratio/proportion:

$$\frac{12.5 \text{ parts}}{70 \text{ parts (total)}} = \frac{x \text{ mls}}{79.2 \text{ ml (TAV from #11)}}$$

Solve for x:

$$70x = 990$$
$$x = 14.14 \text{ ml of Dextrose } 70\% \leftarrow \text{answer #2}$$

We've finished the hard part. The rest is simple ratio/proportion.

- We need 6 meq of Sodium Chloride.

The bottle says the sodium chloride concentration is 4 meq/ml.

Set it up as a ratio/proportion:

$$\frac{4 \text{ meq}}{1 \text{ ml}} = \frac{6 \text{ meq}}{x \text{ ml}}$$

Solve for x:

$$6 = 4x$$
$$x = 1.5 \text{ ml Sodium Chloride} \leftarrow \text{answer to #3}$$

- We need 2.8 meq of Potassium Phosphate.

The bottle says the Potassium Phosphate concentration is 4.4 meq/ml.

Set it up as a ratio/proportion:

$$\frac{4.4 \text{ meq}}{1 \text{ ml}} = \frac{2.8 \text{ meq}}{x \text{ ml}}$$

Solve for x:

$$2.8 = 4.4x$$
$$x = 0.64 \text{ ml Potassium Phosphate} \leftarrow \text{answer to #4}$$

- We need 2 meq of Potassium Chloride.

The bottle says the Potassium Chloride concentration is 2 meq/ml.

Set it up as a ratio/proportion:

$$\frac{2 \text{ meq}}{1 \text{ ml}} = \frac{2 \text{ meq}}{x \text{ ml}}$$

Solve for x:

$$2 = 2x$$
$$x = 1.0 \text{ ml Potassium Chloride} \leftarrow \text{answer to #5}$$

- We need 3 meq of Magnesium Sulfate.

The bottle says the Magnesium Sulfate concentration is 4.06 meq/ml.

Set it up as a ratio/proportion:

$$\frac{4.06 \text{ meq}}{1 \text{ ml}} = \frac{3 \text{ meq}}{x \text{ ml}}$$

Solve for x:

$$3 = 4.06x$$

$$x = 0.74 \text{ ml Magnesium Sulfate} \leftarrow \text{answer to \#6}$$

- We need 3.2 meq of Calcium Gluconate.
  The bottle says the Calcium Gluconate concentration is
  0.47 meq/ml.

Set it up as a ratio/proportion:

$$\frac{0.47 \text{ meq}}{1 \text{ ml}} = \frac{3.3 \text{ meq}}{x \text{ ml}}$$

Solve for x:

$$3.2 = 0.47x$$

$$x = 6.8 \text{ ml Calcium Gluconate} \leftarrow \text{answer to \#7}$$

- We need 6.5 ml of pediatric MVI.
  The TPN order states how many mls need to be added.
  6.5 ml $\leftarrow$ answer to \#8

We need 0.5 units/ml TAV. This translates as 0.5 unit of heparin for every ml that is in the TPN. What is the TAV? 79.2 ml. What are we solving for? How many units are needed?
Set this up as an R/P:

$$\frac{0.5 \text{ units}}{1 \text{ ml}} = \frac{x \text{ units}}{79.2 \text{ ml}}$$

Solve for x:

$$79.2(0.5) = x$$

$$x = 39.6 \text{ units} \leftarrow \text{answer to \#9}$$

Now, figure out how many mls need to be added.

- Heparin comes as 100 units/ml. We need 39.6 units.

Set this up as another R/P:

$$\frac{100 \text{ units}}{1 \text{ ml}} = \frac{39.6 \text{ units}}{x \text{ ml}}$$

Solve for x:

$$39.6 = 100x$$

$$x = 0.39 \text{ ml} \leftarrow \text{answer to \#10}$$

- We need 0.1 ml of Trace Elements.
  The TPN order states how many mls need to be added.
  5.72 ml $\leftarrow$ answer to \#11
- L. The purpose of SWFI is to QS the TPN to the TAV, in this case
  79.2 ml $\leftarrow$ answer to \#12

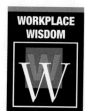

WORKPLACE WISDOM

Heparin will always be a two-part problem to solve to get the correct answer.

Add the additives together (Table 11-2). The difference between the additives and the TAV is the amount of SWFI that must be added.

TABLE 11-2 Calculating the Amount of SWFI

Components	Amount Required	Amount to be added (mls)
Amino Acid (Trophamine 6%)	2.5 gm	1. 41.67 ml
Dextrose 70%	12.5%	2. 14.14 ml
Sodium Chloride	6 meq	3. 1.5 ml
Potassium Phosphate	2.8 meq	4. 0.64 ml
Potassium Chloride	2 meq	5. 1.0 ml
Magnesium Sulfate	3 meq	6. 0.74 ml
Calcium Gluconate	3.2 meq	7. 6.8 ml
Pediatric MVI	6.5 ml	8. 6.5 ml
Heparin	0.5 unit/ml of TAV	9. 39.6 units
Trace Elements	0.1 ml	10. 0.39 ml
SWFI	_____	11. 5.72 ml
TAV	(Total Actual Volume)	12. 79.2 ml

The additives add up to 73.48 ml.

$$\text{TAV} - \text{Additives} = \text{SWFI}$$
$$79.2 - 73.48 = 5.72 \text{ mls SWFI}$$

CHAPTER REVIEW QUESTIONS

SMALL VOLUME PROBLEMS

1. An IV bag, NS 250 mls, is running at a rate of 50 mls/hr. How long should this IV bag last?

2. An IV bag, D5$\frac{1}{2}$NS 500 mls, is running at a rate of 20 mls/hr. How long will this IV bag last?

3. An IV bag, $\frac{1}{2}$NS 1000 mls, is running at a rate of 250 ml/hr. How long should this IV bag last?

4. Gammar PIV 825 mls is running at a rate of 75 ml/hr. How long will this special preparation last?

5. An epidural cassette has a total volume of 200 mls. It is being infused at a rate of 8 ml/hr. How long will this epidural last?

LARGE VOLUME PROBLEMS

6. A 1000 ml bag of D5$\frac{1}{4}$w/20 meq of KCl was hung at 2 P.M. on 11/28/03. If this IV bag is running at a rate of 100 ml/hr, what time should the next bag be hung?

7. If an IV is running at a rate of 125 ml/hr, how many 1000 ml bags will be needed for a 24-hour period?

8. A physician has written an order for a patient to receive 500 ml of IV fluid every 24 hours. What is the rate of this IV?

9. A physician has written an order for a patient to receive 4000 ml of IV fluid every 24 hours. What is the rate of this IV?

Resources and References

1. Ballington, Don. *Pharmacy Practice for Technicians*. EMC Paradigm, 2003.

2. Wilroy, Liz Johnson and Daniel E. Garcia. *Pharmacy Sterile Products Training Manual*. Pharmacy Education Resources 2002. Houston, TX.

3. ASHP website *www.ashp.org*

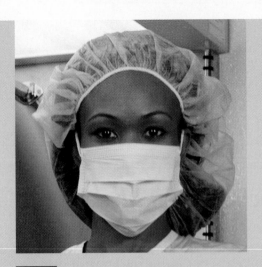

CHAPTER

12

Introduction to Sterile Products

Learning Objectives

After completing this chapter, you should be able to:

- List the necessary equipment and supplies used in preparing sterile products.
- List the routes of administration associated with sterile products.
- Discuss special concerns regarding chemotherapy and cytotoxic drugs.

INTRODUCTION

As pharmacy practice moves to a more patient-centered concept of pharmaceutical care, pharmacists rely on new and expanded roles for pharmacy technicians.

Technicians have assumed many of the drug distribution responsibilities traditionally performed by pharmacists in order to free pharmacists to provide direct patient care. Technicians need to be properly trained and highly qualified to perform these responsibilities. This chapter presents an introduction for pharmacy technicians to sterile products and aseptic technique.

Compounding medications for patients' specific needs is an integral part of the 5,000-year history of pharmacy. As recently as 1938, when the Food, Drug, and Cosmetic Act was introduced, 50 percent of prescriptions were compounded. During that time, pharmacists did most of the drug preparation and distribution. Today, as pharmacists become part of a multidisciplinary, multiskilled team to provide quality patient care, they rely more and more on pharmacy technicians. Technicians have now assumed many of the duties that were once performed by the pharmacist. One such duty is drug preparation, specifically, compounding and intravenous drug preparation.

The term compounding refers to the sterile and nonsterile preparation of many types of made-to-order suspensions, capsules, suppositories, topically applied medications, intravenous admixtures, and parenteral nutrition solutions. Nonsterile compounding includes the first four forms of drug preparation just listed: suspensions, capsules, suppositories, and topicals.

The more complex the compounding becomes, the more precautions and steps will need to be added to guidelines to provide proper aseptic technique.

Aseptic Technique

Aseptic technique is carrying out a procedure under controlled conditions in a manner that minimizes the chance of contamination. What can cause contamination? Contamination can be caused by the following factors:

environment—controlling the air where the compounding is being performed

equipment—all objects that come in contact with the drug(s) must be sterile

personnel—touch contamination is the most frequent cause of contamination

We will address each of these causes of contamination in detail, since each plays a key role in proper aseptic compounding. The preparation of sterile drug compounds requires the utmost diligence to ensure final product integrity and sterility. Sterile products must be prepared with aseptic technique in a class 100 environment. This is a classification of an airflow unit capable of producing an environment containing no more than 100 airborne particles of a size 0.5 micron and larger, per cubic foot of air. Such an environment exists inside a certified horizontal or vertical laminar flow hood, a class 100 clean room, and a barrier isolator. A barrier isolator is a closed system made up of four solid walls, an air-handling system, and a transfer and interaction compartment.

Basic Equipment and Supplies

Basic equipment and supplies include laminar flow hoods, vertical flow hoods, biological safety cabinets, needles, syringes, and IV bags.

LAMINAR FLOW HOODS

Laminar flow hoods are designed to reduce the risk of airborne contamination during the preparation of IV admixtures by providing an ultra-clean environment. The most important part of a laminar flow hood is a high-efficiency, bacteria-retentive filter, commonly called a HEPA (high-efficiency particulate air) filter. Room air is taken into the unit and passed through a prefilter to remove relatively large contaminants such as dust and lint. The air is then compressed and channeled up behind and through the HEPA filter, where virtually all bacteria are removed. The purified air then flows out over the entire work surface in parallel lines at a uniform velocity.

A laminar flow hood has three basic functions. The first is to provide clean air in the working area. This is done by passing room air through a bacteria-retentive filter to provide a continuous flow of clean air in the work area. Second, the constant flow of air out of the laminar flow hood prevents room air from entering the work area. Last, the air flowing out suspends and removes contaminants introduced into the work area by material (such as IV bags, syringes, and drug packaging) or personnel. Thus, a laminar flow hood provides an environment virtually free of airborne contaminants, in which procedures can be safely performed.

Laminar flow hoods may be used in the pharmacy to perform the following procedures:

- preparation of IV admixtures
- preparation of ophthalmic solutions
- reconstitution of powdered drugs
- filling unit dose syringes
- preparation of miscellaneous sterile products

Laminar flow hoods come in various sizes and models. One model, called a console model, sits on the floor. The other common model is called a bench or countertop model, because it sits on top of the counter, and the space underneath it can be used for storage space. Laminar airflow hoods are usually kept running continuously. If the hood is turned off, it is recommended to run it for at least 30 minutes before using the work surface area in order to replace the room air with clean, filtered air. Laminar flow hoods should be inspected and certified every six months to assure that the HEPA filter is intact, unclogged, and has no holes in it. The prefilters in the hoods should be changed monthly. (See Figure 12-1.)

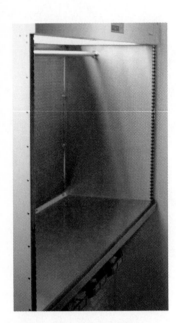

Figure 12-1 Laminar airflow hood

VERTICAL FLOW HOODS

Both the console and bench models are available with vertical rather than horizontal airflow. With vertical flow, room air enters at the top of the unit and is channeled through the bacteria-retentive filter (which forms the ceiling of the unit) and down vertically across the work surface area. Neither of these models of laminar flow hoods should be used when preparing chemotherapy drugs. Although they protect the drug product from microbial contamination, they do not protect personnel or the environment from the hazards of the drug agents. These laminar flow hoods blow air across the work surface toward the operator and into the work environment. Drug particles or aerosols of these hazardous agents can easily contaminate both workers and the work environment.

BIOLOGICAL SAFETY CABINETS

Rather than a horizontal laminar flow hood, a biological safety cabinet is recommended to provide protection for the worker, the work environment, and the drug. Figure 12-2 shows what a biological safety cabinet looks like.

A biological safety cabinet functions by having air taken into the unit at the top, where it passes through a prefilter to remove large contaminants. Air then passes through a HEPA filter and is directed down toward the work surface, just as with a vertical laminar flow hood. The filter forms the ceiling of the work area in the biological safety cabinet and removes bacteria to provide ultraclean air. Unlike the mechanism in a vertical laminar flow hood, however, as air approaches the work surface, it is pulled through vents at the front, back, and sides of the unit. A major portion of the contaminated air is recirculated back into the cabinet, and a minor portion is passed through a HEPA filter before being exhausted into the room.

Biological safety cabinets are of two basic types. A Class 2, type A, which was just described, represents the minimum recommended environment for preparing chemotherapy agents. Class 2, type B biological safety cabinets have greater intake flow velocities and are vented outside the building rather than back into the room. This type of safety cabinet is preferred, but the need to vent the filtered air to the outside can carry with it a substantial construction cost.

It is important that biological safety cabinets run continuously. If turned off for any reason, such as for maintenance or changing the HEPA filter, the biological safety cabinet must be thoroughly cleaned with a detergent, and the exhaust area must be covered with impermeable plastic and sealed to prevent any contaminants from escaping from the unit.

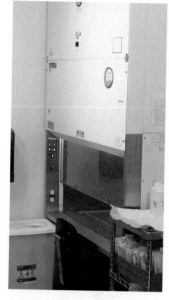

Figure 12-2   Biological safety cabinet

NEEDLES

A needle consists of two parts: the shaft and the hub. The shaft is the long, slender stem of the needle that is beveled (diagonal cut) at one end to form a point. The hollow bore of the needle shaft is known as the lumen. At the other end of the needle is the hub, to which a syringe can be attached. (See Figure 12-3.)

Needle size is designated by length and gauge. The length of a needle is measured in inches from the juncture of the hub and the shaft to the tip of the point. Needle lengths range from $\frac{3}{8}$ inch to $3\frac{1}{2}$ inch or longer. The gauge of a needle, used to designate the size of the lumen, ranges from 27, the finest, to 13, the largest. The finer the needle, the higher the gauge number will be. In some disposable needles, the gauge is designated by color of the hub (in order to facilitate recognition). One factor in choosing a needle size is the thickness (viscosity) of the injectable solution. A fine needle with a relatively small lumen may be acceptable for most solutions, but a needle with a larger lumen and a smaller gauge number may be needed for more viscous solutions. Another factor in selecting the proper needle is the nature of the rubber closure to be penetrated. A fine needle with a smaller lumen may be preferred for rubber closures that core easily, meaning that part of the rubber closure gets carried into the drug solution when the needle penetrates the rubber closure. Needles are sterilized, individually wrapped, and disposable. Never reuse a used needle.

Filter needles are similar to other needles, except that they have a filter in the hub to catch any particles from an ampule or vial and are used to vent small-volume vials.

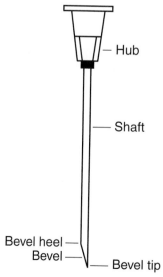

Figure 12-3   Parts of a needle

Dispensing pins are just one example of the various styles that are available from the many different distributors out there. Each works in the same fashion by providing a venting system to trap any particles larger than its pores. There are a variety of different pore sizes available. A 0.22 micron pore size is considered to be a sterilizing filter capable of removing all microorganisms. Other sizes commonly used in the pharmacy and suitable for clarifying solutions have a porosity of 0.45, 1, 5, or 10 micron. Picking one over another depends upon your ability to manipulate the pin and the cost of the device.

SYRINGES

The two basic parts of a syringe are the barrel and the plunger (Figure 12-4). The barrel is a tube that is open at one end, tapering into a hollow tip at the other end. The open end is extended radically outward to form a rim, or flange, to prevent the barrel from slipping through the fingers during manipulation.

The plunger is a piston-type rod with a slightly cone-shaped tip that passes inside the barrel of the syringe. The other end of the plunger is shaped into a flat knob for easy manipulation. The plunger must be able to move freely throughout the barrel, yet its surface must be so close to the barrel that the fluid cannot pass in between, even when under considerable pressure.

The tip of the syringe provides the point of attachment for a needle. The tip may be tapered to allow the needle hub to be slipped over it and held on by friction. When this method is used, the needle is reasonably secure, but it may slip off if not properly attached or if considerable pressure is used to inject the solution. Locking devices have been developed to secure the needle more firmly on the tip of the syringe; one such device has the trade name Luer-Lok. These devices incorporate a collar with a circular internal groove into which the needle hub is inserted. A half-turn locks the needle in place. This method is especially valuable when pressure is required.

Graduation lines on the barrel of the syringe indicate the volume of solution inside. Accurate readings are more easily made if the color of the tip of the plunger is different from that of the syringe itself. Syringes are disposable

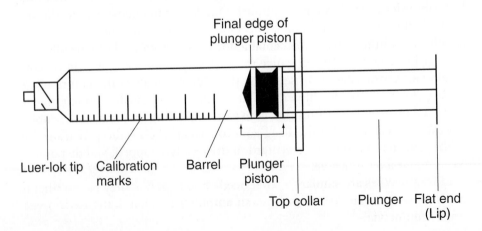

Figure 12-4 Parts of a syringe

and have a capacity range of 1–60 ml. Graduation lines may be in milliliter, depending on the capacity of the syringe; for example, the larger the capacity of the syringe, the larger is the interval between graduation lines. Special-purpose syringes, such as insulin syringes, have graduation lines in both milliliters and insulin units to reflect their intended use.

In the selection of an appropriate syringe, as a rule the capacity of the syringe should be the next size larger than the volume to be measured. For example, a 3 ml syringe should be selected to measure a 2.3 ml dose, or a 5 ml syringe to measure a 3.8 ml dose. In this way, the graduation marks on the syringe will be in the smallest possible increments for the dose measured. Syringes should not be filled to capacity, because the plunger can easily be dislodged. It is recommended that syringes containing chemotherapy drugs not be filled more than three-quarters of capacity.

Sterile, disposable syringes are discarded after one use and have the same advantages as disposable needles. Although syringes today are made of plastic because it costs less, glass syringes can still be bought for drugs that are incompatible with plastic. Syringes and needles need to be disposed of in a sharps container. Do not recap needles after they have been used.

Some pharmaceutical manufacturers supply common doses of frequently used or emergency-use drugs in prefilled syringes. Prefilled syringes eliminate the need to measure doses, thus saving valuable time in compounding admixtures. Prefilled syringes are commonly seen in emergency carts or are used in emergency rooms when it is critical to get the medication to the patient as quickly as possible. Some pharmaceutical manufacturers supply common doses of frequently used drugs in prefilled syringes. Prefilled syringes eliminate the need to measure doses, thus saving valuable time in compounding admixtures.

Most prefilled syringes are supplied in a syringe that does not have a plunger. This is to prevent the drug from accidentally squirting out if pressure were applied to the plunger when being stored or transferred. A device called a tubex holder is screwed onto the back of the syringe (where the plunger would have been), and a locking ring is then tightened around the end of the syringe.

IV BAGS

Plastic bags are used for diluting a solution and are the most common way of administering intravenous medications to patients. Plastic bags are available in many different sizes, with 50, 100, 250, 500, and 1000 ml being the most common. Special bags for compounding parenteral nutrition are available in 2,000 ml and 3,000 ml sizes. Some IV bags are made of PVC (polyvinyl chloride). More expensive than plastic bags, these bags are used for specific drugs (like Taxol) that can adhere to the plastic of the non-PVC IV bags. Figure 12-5 shows the two types of IV bags that are commonly used.

At the top of the bag is a flat plastic extension with a hole to allow it to be hung on an administration pole. At the other end of the bag are two ports of about the same length. The administration set port has a blue plastic cover that serves to maintain the sterility of the port. The cover is easily removed

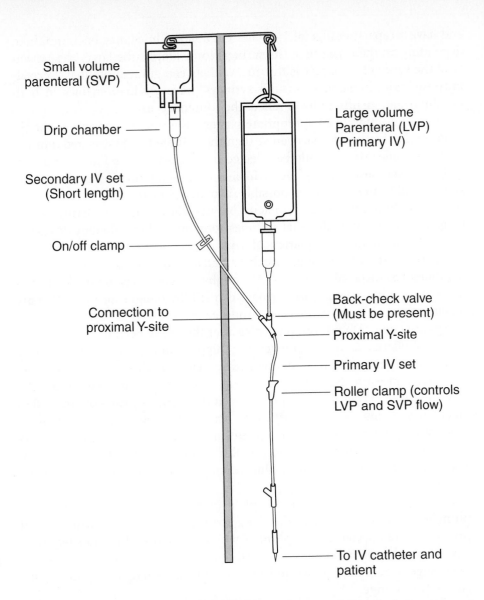

Small volume parenteral (SVP)

Drip chamber

Secondary IV set (Short length)

On/off clamp

Connection to proximal Y-site

Large volume Parenteral (LVP) (Primary IV)

Back-check valve (Must be present)

Proximal Y-site

Primary IV set

Roller clamp (controls LVP and SVP flow)

To IV catheter and patient

Figure 12-5 Components of an IV bag and tubing

by pulling on it. Once it is pulled off, the sterile port of the administration set is exposed. Solution will not drip from the plastic bag at this point because a plastic diaphragm about $\frac{1}{2}$ inch inside the port seals in the liquid. The spike of the administration set is inserted into the port, puncturing the inner diaphragm to allow the solution to flow from the flexible plastic bag into the administration set. When the solution has filled the administration set (this process is called "priming" the set), make sure to clamp the administration set so that the solution does not leak out. Once the inner diaphragm is punctured, it is not resealable.

The other port is the medication port. It is covered by a protective rubber tip. Medication is added to the solution through the medication port by means of a needle and syringe. The rubber tip is self-sealing, thus preventing solution from leaking when the needle punctures the tip. Approximately $\frac{1}{2}$ inch inside this port is a plastic diaphragm that must be punctured for solution to enter the bag. The inner diaphragm is not self-sealing when punctured by a needle, so the rubber tip must stay attached to the bag. Graduation marks to indicate the volume of solution infused are located on both sides of the front of some plastic bags at 25–100 ml intervals, depending on their capacity.

When you place a label on a plastic bag, it does not matter which side of the bag you place the label; however, many institutions place the label on the printed side of the bag, beneath the solution name, and offset slightly to one side so that the graduation marks near the side can still be read. This procedure has the advantage of providing a convenient cross-check between the actual solution and the name appearing on the admixture label.

Some IV solutions, such as 5 percent dextrose injection and 0.9 percent sodium chloride injection, are available in minibags, or piggyback bags. These bags typically hold 50 ml or 100 ml of solution and are used to administer drugs (such as antibiotics) intermittently rather than continuously.

The plastic bag system is completely closed to air. It does not depend on air to displace the solution as it leaves the bag. The bag collapses as the solution is administered, so a vacuum is not created inside.

Routes of Administration

When drugs need to be injected, any one of several routes can be used to administer the drug. Often, certain drugs can be administered only through specific routes, and this will be listed in the package insert. The most common injectable routes of administration are intravenous (in the vein), intramuscular (in the muscle), and subcutaneous (in the skin). There are other, less used routes that include intradermal (in the dermis of the skin), and intrathecal (in the spine).

Intravenous administration of drugs has advantages over other routes because it provides the fastest route to the bloodstream. There are no barriers like skin or muscle to absorb the drug first, which will allow the most rapid onset of action. If someone cannot take medication by mouth because he is unconscious or vomiting, then intravenous administration is the best route. Since the inner lining of a vein is relatively insensitive to pain, drugs that can be irritating if given by another route can be given intravenously at a slow rate without causing pain. Drugs that can be diluted to reduce irritation can be given only intravenously, because the tissues around the other routes cannot accommodate the large volume.

RISKS

There are some risks involved in intravenous administration. One risk is that, if there is an error in the dose, the drug is difficult to stop it because it is very quickly dispersed throughout the body and will start working within a few minutes. Another risk is the possibility of infection anytime the skin is punctured. This risk demands the knowledge and skills to prepare sterile products to reduce the chance of infection to the patient.

INTRAVENOUS ADMINISTRATION

There are two types of intravenous administration. The first is an intravenous injection in which the prepared medication is drawn up into a syringe and administered over a short time. The amount of medication is usually a small volume pushed through an IV line that is already in place on the patient. Before a medication is pushed into the vein, the syringe is pulled slightly back to draw blood out or aspirated to make sure that the tip of the needle is in the vein.

The second type of administration is an IV infusion. Infusions are given to overcome dehydration, to build up depleted blood volumes, and to serve as an aid for the administration of medications. An infusion allows a larger volume of solution to be given at a constant rate, depending on the drug to be administered. Infusions can be administered continuously or intermittently. Continuous infusions are used to administer larger volumes of solutions over several hours at a slow, constant rate. Intermittent infusions are used to administer a relatively small volume over a short time at specific intervals.

Sterile Products

Certain characteristics are desired in an IV solution. Some of the characteristics can be seen by visual inspection, and others cannot. The solution must be clear, which should not be confused with colorless, to indicate that the drug added is completely dissolved. IV fat emulsions that are mostly used in conjunction with TPNs are an exception to this rule, because they look similar to milk. A solution must also be free of any visible particulate matter (such as rubber cores from vials).

STERILITY

Sterility is the freedom from bacteria and other microorganisms. Solutions to be injected must be sterile. A product is either sterile or not sterile; products cannot be partially sterile. Sterility cannot be visibly seen, but proper aseptic technique can maintain the sterility of solutions, drugs, and supplies during preparation.

pH

The term pH is used to describe the degree of acidity of a solution. pH values range from 0 to 14, with values below 7 representing greater acidity of the solution, while values above 7 represent less acidity or greater alkalinity. A solution having a pH of 7 is neither acidic nor alkaline; it is considered neutral. Plasma in our body is about 7.4, and solutions should try to stay around that number. pH is another characteristic that cannot be seen, but can be tested after it is prepared.

TONICITY

A final characteristic that also cannot be seen is isotonicity. An isotonic solution has the same concentration as red blood cells. Isotonic IV solutions minimize patient discomfort and damage to red blood cells. Stinging caused by either a hypertonic (shrinking of red blood cells) or hypotonic (swelling of red blood cells) solution is not experienced with an isotonic solution. IV solutions should be as close to isotonic as possible. A good reference point to remember is that 0.9 percent sodium chloride injection and 5 percent dextrose injection are both approximately isotonic.

STORAGE

When storing sterile products, try to avoid places that are exposed to extreme hot or cold temperatures. Exposing products to cold temperatures could cause some drugs in the solution to precipitate. Solutions that contain drugs should also not be exposed to high temperatures because such storage may accelerate decomposition of the drug. IV solutions should be kept at room temperature or in a cool place.

COMMON PRODUCTS

There are many different types of solutions commercially available; however, three types are most frequently used: sodium chloride injection, dextrose injection, and Ringer's injection. These three most resemble the plasma in our blood. Sodium chloride 0.9 percent and dextrose 5 percent are isotonic, as mentioned earlier, but both provide a source of fluid and electrolyte replacement. Ringer's injection can be modified with the addition of sodium lactate to produce lactated Ringer's injection. Ringer's solutions are primarily used for fluid replacement and as a source of electrolytes.

COMPATIBILITY

Not all drugs are compatible with each other. The incompatibility may be between two drugs or between a drug and an IV solution. The possibility of an unexpected or undesirable combination is relatively low compared with the number of IV admixtures prepared, but it is always possible. An incompatibility can lead to a patient not receiving the full therapeutic dose of a medication or, even worse, can lead to an adverse reaction. Some incompatibilities, such as a color change or hazy appearance, can be seen. Precipitate can form in the solution, or an evolution of a gas may even be smelled. Be aware that sometimes when drugs are combined and a visible change occurs, it could be expected and harmless. Reading the package insert or checking with the pharmacist can confirm the reason for this change in appearance. Other incompatibilities cannot be visually recognized. If two drugs are mixed that are incompatible with each other, one drug can cause the degradation of the other drug. Many factors can affect the compatibility and stability of drugs in IV admixtures. The following list describes each of the factors:

- pH—pH is one of the most common causes of incompatibilities. Combining two drugs that require two different pH values for the final solution can cause one or both drugs to either degrade or precipitate.
- Light—Some drugs will start to break down and lose their therapeutic effect if exposed to light.
- Dilution—the concentration of a drug in solution may be a factor in its compatibility with other drugs. A problem can be avoided by assuring that the drug in question is properly diluted before it is combined with the other drug.
- Chemical composition—the chemical complexity of one drug can cause a reduced therapeutic effect of the other drug, because when the two drugs combine, their new chemical combination may initiate adverse events.
- Time—Most drugs start to degrade in a short time after being added to an IV solution.
- Solutions—Some drugs require a specific solution or diluent to be used for reconstitution and further dilution. Choosing the wrong solution can cause the drug to be broken down more quickly or can cause precipitate to form. Some drugs are packaged with a specific diluent for reconstitution; an example of this is Herceptin (Trastuzumab).
- Temperature—Heat increases the rate of most chemical reactions, and since the degradation of a drug in solution can be considered a chemical reaction, care must be taken to keep admixtures at a stable temperature. Some drugs can remain more stable refrigerated than if they were kept at room temperature. Some drugs, however, should never be refrigerated because a precipitate can form. Not many experts recommend freezing drugs after reconstitution, and sometimes freezing actually reduces the stability of the drug.
- Buffer capacity—This is the ability of a solution to resist a change in pH when either an acidic or alkaline substance is added to the solution. Many drugs contain buffers to increase their stability. IV solutions in general do not have high buffer capacities. So, when a drug with a high buffer capacity is added, the resulting solution will have a pH closest to the drug added.
- Order of Mixing—The order in which drugs are added to the solution may be a factor in compatibility. Drugs that are concentrated and combined may react to form precipitate, whereas both drugs in diluted solutions may be combined acceptably. This is very important when mixing parenteral nutrition solutions (which will be discussed in detail later). Electrolytes are commonly prescribed with phosphates, and this causes a mixing problem when mixing parenteral solutions if it is not done correctly. To avoid the problem, it is important to mix the solution well after each addition is made and then to add the electrolytes last after the phosphate has been well diluted.

- Plastic—As mentioned earlier, some drugs are incompatible with the plastic container that the solution will be placed in. Polyvinyl chloride (PVC) plastic can leach certain properties of the plastic out of the bag, or the drug may adhere to the bag. It is recommended that one use a non-PVC container for these specific drugs.
- Filters—Filters were also mentioned earlier and represent a possible problem in effectively administering a drug to a patient. Filters can cause a reduction in concentration of the drug to be administered.

To minimize incompatibilities, the following general guidelines need to be followed whenever possible:

1. Use solutions promptly after preparation in order to ensure administration of the most stable product; drugs tend to degrade in a relatively short time. If a newly made admixture is not immediately used, it should be placed in the refrigerator.

2. Minimize the number of drugs added to a solution. As the number of drugs added increases, the chance of an incompatibility rises. It becomes increasingly difficult to find information on compatibilities when more than two drugs are added to a solution.

3. Check incompatibility resources to verify which drugs have a very high or very low pH. Since most drugs are acidic, their combination with a drug having a very high pH is more likely to result in an incompatibility.

The most often used resources for information on incompatibilities are the manufacturers' drug package inserts. The package inserts have a wealth of information about the drug. The package insert is developed by the manufacturer and approved by the FDA (Food & Drug Administration) when the drug is marketed. The package insert generally isn't as great of a reference for incompatibilities specifically; however, there are other excellent resources out there, like incompatibility charts, articles in professional magazines, reference books, and the Internet that can give you more accurate and up-to-date information. Incompatibility charts list drugs that can and cannot be mixed in particular solutions. Some charts list drugs horizontally across the top and vertically down one side. One drug is found in the top list and the other drug in the side list; then the two constituents of the admixture are followed along the lines from the top and the side until they intersect. A notation in the space where the lines intersect denotes whether the mixture is compatible. (One problem with this kind of chart is that it does not list the reason the two drugs are incompatible.)

The American Journal of Health-System Pharmacy frequently has detailed research articles on intravenous incompatibilities. Some very useful reference books are the *Handbook of Injectable Drugs* and the *Facts and Comparisons Book*. Many pharmacy departments maintain a file that categorizes drugs to make looking up drug information quicker and easier. Some pharmacy computer systems screen IV admixture incompatibilities as well as drug interactions, alerting the pharmacist or pharmacy technician to these issues when the order is entered, before it is prepared.

TPNs—TOTAL PARENTERAL NUTRITION

Parenteral nutrition solutions are complex admixtures used to provide nutritional support to patients who are unable to take in adequate nutrients through the gastrointestinal tract. These admixtures are composed of such things as fat, protein, dextrose, electrolytes, vitamins, and water. Parenteral solutions can be formulated and calculated to match an individual's nutritional requirements. Parenteral nutrition solutions are also referred to as TPN solutions. Due to the complexity and time needed to prepare a TPN solution, many pharmacies that compound a large number of parenteral nutrition solutions use high-speed compounders, Automixers, or Micromixers. These machines prepare complex solutions safely, accurately, and quickly. Automixers can hold from two to ten different components of the appropriate solution to be mixed.

These compounders consist of two principal parts: the pump module and the control module. The pump module is placed in the laminar flow hood along with the components that hang from hangers in the hood. A disposable transfer set is hooked up to the machine, and then each tubing, or lead, is inserted into each component. Each lead is color coded to its specific spot on the compounder. All the leads come together at a junction and are connected to the final solution that is hanging from a hanger hooked up to an electronic scale that measures fluid by weight. This way is more accurate than measuring fluid volume because it is not adversely affected by air entering the system.

The control module is the computer that controls how much of each component will be needed for the final solution. It is kept outside the laminar flow hood and is controlled by using the keypad to enter data for each component. Some pharmacies have installed a bar code system to their automixers to detect when a lead is not correctly attached to the right station. The bar code is scanned against the lead tubing and then scanned at the corresponding station; if they match the correct attachment is assured. If the bar codes don't match when scanned, then an alarm sounds and an error display appears on the control module.

Parenteral nutrition solutions need to be administered with caution. There are two ways to administer parenteral nutrition solutions intravenously. The first is through a central vein, and the second is through a peripheral vein. They are most commonly infused into a large central vein that leads directly to the heart. The subclavian vein, under the collarbone, is used most often.

CHEMOTHERAPY

The use of chemotherapy or antineoplastics to treat cancer began in the late 1940s. It was not until the late 1970s that health professionals became aware of potential hazards associated with the handling of antineoplastic drugs. Concern has been steadily mounting over the risks incurred by pharmacy staff that prepare and dispose of cytotoxic agents. Most of these agents were designed to damage the DNA of rapidly dividing cancer cells. However, because they lack specificity, any rapidly dividing cells in the body, whether normal or cancerous, become damaged. Repeated exposure to DNA-active drugs over a long period of time could potentially lead to irreparable DNA damage and some mutations, whether cancerous or not, to occur to unborn babies.

Health problems caused by acute exposure to cytotoxic agents include sensitivity, coughing, dizziness, headaches, caustic vesicant-like marks, and eye reactions. These can occur by direct skin contact, inhalation, ingestion, or accidental injection of agents. The long-term consequences of low-dose exposure to antineoplastic agents are also a serious concern. There is no conclusive proof that exists to date that the potential problems associated with preparing these drugs will occur in professionals who have minimal exposure from handling these products. Furthermore, there is neither a known threshold of danger nor a reliable method of monitoring exposure to health care workers.

Several agencies, including the Occupational Safety and Health Administration (OSHA), the National Institutes of Health (NIH), and the American Society of Health System Pharmacists (ASHP) have issued guidelines regarding the safe handling of drugs. Common sense dictates that, regardless of the type or size of the facility, practical solutions are necessary for employee protection. Any organization handling cancer chemotherapy or other hazardous drugs must accept the following standards as essential components of occupational safety:

- written policies and procedures
- employee education
- certification
- continuing education
- proper aseptic technique
- access to medical attention for employees exposed to hazardous drugs
- appropriate documentation of exposure incidents

Employees must be informed of the possible risks and controversies at the time of hire and should be given the option of reassignment at vulnerable periods in their lives. For women, these may include documented pregnancy and breast-feeding. Some pregnant personnel choose to continue handling chemotherapeutic agents because they are confident that their workplace provides adequate protection. Some men may request a transfer away from preparing drugs when planning a family because of the possible impact on a male's sperm count.

An employee's competence and understanding of good work practices should be tested not only before hire, but also periodically throughout employment, through observation and written evaluation. Up-to-date policies and procedures for compounding sterile products should be written and available to all personnel involved in IV preparation. When policies and procedures are changed and additions or deletions are made to them, these updates need to be communicated to all employees involved in drug preparation. The policy and procedures should address education and training requirements,

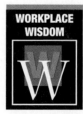

WORKPLACE WISDOM

This chapter is just an overview of this specialty practice in institutional pharmacy. Specific techniques have not been included, as they are too advanced and detailed for the scope of this book. For an in-depth look at sterile products and step-by-step procedures for aseptic technique, review *Sterile Products for Technicians*, published by Prentice Hall Health.

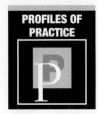
Certain states require pharmacy technicians to be certified in aseptic technique prior to working in the clean-room environment, and some states require technicians working with sterile products to complete a specific number of live, continuing education programs related to aseptic technique each year.

The National Pharmacy Technician Association offers a Sterile Products Certification Course, which is valid nationwide and meets the most stringent of state requirements. In addition, NPTA offers live CE programs to aid technicians. For more information on either of these offers, contact NPTA via the web at *www.pharmacytechnician.org* or by calling 1-888-247-8700.

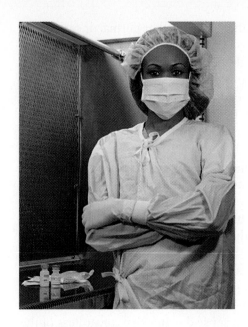

Figure 12-6
IV technician

competency evaluations, storage and handling of products and supplies, storage and delivery of final products, maintenance of facilities and equipment used in the preparation, appropriate garments worn, validation of proper preparation technique, labeling of final products, documentation, quality control, and conduct for personnel working in the controlled area. (See Figure 12-6.)

CONCLUSION

Sterile product preparation can be a complex, high-risk process in the healthcare setting. Pharmacy technicians play an integral role in the procurement, storage, preparation, and distribution of these products. Training, education, and measuring competency are critical to assure a safe chemotherapy process for patients and for employees. Increasing pharmacy technicians' awareness of safety standards for preparing sterile products will ensure a safe work environment and reduce potential medication errors.

CHAPTER 12

CHAPTER REVIEW QUESTIONS

1. The following are the basic functions of the air flow in a laminar flow hood, except:
   a. prevent room air from entering the hood
   b. provide clean air in the hood
   c. suspend and remove contaminants introduced into the hood
   d. provide personnel with protection from hazardous agents

2. Laminar flow hoods may be used to perform the following procedures, except:
   a. reconstitution of powdered drugs
   b. preparation of ophthalmic solutions
   c. preparation of hazardous drugs
   d. filling unit-dose syringes

3. What does HEPA stand for?
   a. Huge Effective Particulate Aerolizer
   b. High Efficiency Particulate Air
   c. Highly Effective Particulate Air
   d. High Efficiency Particular Airborne

4. What micron pore size is considered to be a sterilizing filter?
   a. 0.45
   b. 0.22
   c. 5
   d. 1

5. Which route of administration is given in the vein?
   a. intramuscular
   b. intradermal
   c. intrathecal
   d. intravenous

6. The desired characteristics of an intravenous solution include:
   a. sterile
   b. colorless
   c. clear (except fat emulsions)
   d. free of particulate

7. When an intravenous solution is considered neutral, what is its pH?
   a. 0
   b. 7
   c. 14
   d. 7.4

8. The following are factors that can affect compatibility or stability of drugs, except:
   a. strength of the drug
   b. dilution of the drug in a solution
   c. chemical composition of the drug with another drug
   d. pH of the drug with another drug

9. The following are the essential components of occupational safety for any organization, except:
   a. proper aseptic technique
   b. continuing education
   c. DNA samples from all employees
   d. certification

10. Which of the following is not a form of personal protective equipment?
    a. prescription eyeglasses
    b. gloves
    c. gown
    d. face shield

Resources and References

1. Attolio, Richard M. "Caring Enough to Understand: The Road to Oncology Medication Error Prevention." *Hospital Pharmacy Volume 31.* Philadelphia, PA: Lippincott-Raven Publishers, 1996: 17–26.

2. Ballington, Don A. *Pharmacy Practice for Technicians.* St. Paul: EMC Paradigm Publishing Inc., 1999.

3. Bergemann, Donald A. "Handling Antineoplastic Agents." *The American Journal of Intravenous Therapy and Clinical Nutrition.* Bethesda, MD: ASCN. 1983: 13–17.

4. Blecher, C.S., E.M. Glynn-Tucker, M. McDiarmid, and S.A. Newton, Ed. *Safe Handling of Hazardous Drugs.* Pittsburgh, PA: ONS Publishing. 2003.

5. Buchanan, E. *Sterile Compounding Facilities.* Principles of sterile product preparation. Bethesda, MD: ASPH. 1995: 25–35.

6. Dorr, Robert T. *Practical Safety Precautions for Handling Cytotoxic Agents in Hospital Pharmacies.* Tucson, AZ: The University of Arizona Health Sciences Center, 1990.

7. Hunt, Max L. Jr., Ed. *Training Manual for Intravenous Admixture Personnel.* Chicago: Precept Press, 1995.

8. King, L.D. "Considering Compounding." *America's Pharmacist.* Alexandria, VA: National Community of Pharmacists Association, 2002.

9. Talley, Richard C. "Sterile Compounding in Hospital Pharmacies." *American Journal of Health-System Pharmacists.* Bethesda, MD: 2003.

10. Thompson, Cheryl A. "USP Publishes Enforceable Chapter on Sterile Compounding." *American Journal of Health-System Pharmacists.* Bethesda, MD: 2003.

11. American Society of Health-System Pharmacists. "ASHP Guidelines on Quality Assurance for Pharmacy-Prepared Sterile Products." *American Journal of Health-System Pharmacists.* Bethesda, MD: 2000: 57: 1150–69.

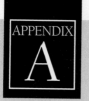

APPENDIX A

Professional Resources

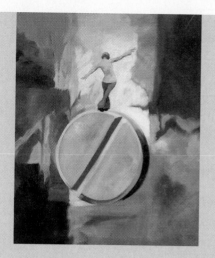

REFERENCE BOOKS

Clinical Books

- *Facts and Comparisons*
- *Drug Handbook for the Allied Health Professional*
- *Martindale's*
- *American Hospital Formulary Service Drug Information, AHFS*
- *Physician's Drug Reference (paid for by drug manufacturers)*

Product Information

- *First Data Bank*
- *American Drug Index*

Pharmaceutical Management

- *The Merck Manual*
- *Manual of Therapeutics*
- *Applied Therapeutics: The Clinical Use of Drugs*

CERTIFICATION, ACCREDITATION, AND REGULATION RESOURCES

PTCB—Pharmacy Technician Certification Board

www.ptcb.org

800-363-8012 (phone)
202-429-7596 (fax)

2215 Constitution Avenue, NW
Washington, DC 20037

PES—Professional Examination Services

www.proexam.org

212-367-4200 phone
212-367-4266 fax

475 Riverside Drive
6th Floor
New York, New York 10115
(They administer the PTCB certification exam.)

ACPE—Accreditation Council for Pharmacy Education

www.acpe-accredit.org

312-664-3575 phone
312-664-4652 fax

20 North Clark Street
Suite 2500
Chicago, Illinois 60602

NABP—National Association of Boards of Pharmacy

www.nabp.net

847-698-6227 phone

700 Busse Highway
Park Ridge, Illinois 60068

NATIONAL ASSOCIATIONS

NPTA—National Pharmacy Technician Association

www.pharmacytechnician.org

888-247-8700 phone
281-895-7320 fax

3707 FM 1960 Road West
Suite 460
Houston, Texas 77068

AAPT—American Association of Pharmacy Technicians

www.pharmacytechnician.com

877-368-4771 phone
336-333-9068 fax

Post Office Box 1447
Greensboro, North Carolina 27402

PTEC—Pharmacy Technician Educators Council

www.rxptec.org

360-992-2817 phone

1800 East McLoughlin Blvd.
Attention: Jeannie Barkett
Vancouver, Washington 98663

CAPT—Canadian Association of Pharmacy Technicians

www.capt.ca

416-410-1142 phone

Post Office Box 1271, Station F
Toronto, Ontario M4Y 2V8

APhA—American Pharmacists Association

www.aphanet.org

202-628-4410 phone

2214 Constitution Avenue, NW
Washington, DC 22037

ASHP—American Society of Health-System Pharmacists

www.ashp.org

301-657-3000 phone

7272 Wisconsin Avenue
Bethesda, Maryland 20814

OTHER RESOURCES

NACDS—National Association of Chain Drug Stores

www.nacds.org

NACP—National Community Pharmacists Association

www.ncpanet.org

FDA—Food & Drug Administration

www.fda.gov

CDC—Centers for Disease Control

www.cdc.gov

APHA—American Public Health Association

www.apha.org

WebMD

www.webmd.com

B

Measurement Charts

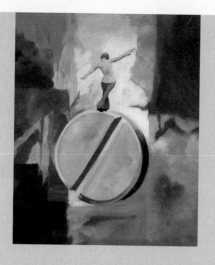

Metric Prefixes with Standard Measures

	Unit	Abbreviation	Equivalents
Weight	**gram**	g or gm	1 g = 1000 mg
	milligram	mg	1 mg = 1000 mcg = 0.001 g
	microgram	mcg	1 mcg = 0.001 mg = 0.000001 g
	kilogram	kg	1 kg = 1000 g
Volume	**liter**	L or l	1 L = 1000 ml
	milliliter	mL or ml	1 ml = 1 cc = 0.001 L
	cubic centimeter	cc	1 cc = 1 ml = 0.001 L
Length	**meter**	m	1 m = 100 cm = 1000 mm
	centimeter	cm	1 cm = 0.01 m = 10 mm
	millimeter	mm	1 mm = 0.001 m = 0.1 cm

Apothecaries' Weights

20 grains (gr)	=	1 scruple		
3 scruples	=	1 dram	=	60 grains
8 drams	=	1 ounce	=	480 grains
12 ounces	=	1 pound	=	5760 grains

Apothecaries' Fluid Measures

60 minims	=	1 fluid dram		
8 fluid drams	=	1 fluid ounce	=	480 minims
16 fluid ounces	=	1 pint		
2 pints	=	1 quart	=	32 fluid ounces
4 quarts	=	1 gallon	=	128 fluid ounces

Avoirdupois Weights

1 ounce (oz)	=	4375 grains (gr)	=	28.4 gm
16 ounces	=	1 pound (lb)	=	7,000 gr

Household Measure Equivalents

3 teaspoonsful (tsp)	=	1 tablespoonful (tbsp)
2 tablespoonsful	=	1 fluid ounce (fl oz)
8 fluid ounces	=	1 cup
2 cups	=	1 pint (pt)
2 pints	=	1 quart (qt)
4 quarts	=	1 gallon (gal)

Household Measures and Metric Conversion Values

1 tsp	=	5 ml
1 tbsp	=	15 ml
1 fl oz	=	30 ml
1 cup	=	240 ml
2.2 lb	=	1 kg
1 ml	=	20 drops (gtt)

Apothecary Measure		Metric Equivalent
15 minims	=	1 ml
1 fluid dram	=	4 ml
1 fluid ounce	=	30 ml
1 ounce	=	8 drams
1 dram	=	60 grains
6 fluid ounces	=	180 ml
8 fluid ounces	=	240 ml
16 fluid ounces	=	500 ml
32 fluid ounces	=	1000 ml
1 grain	=	65 milligrams
1 ounce	=	480 grains
15 grains	=	1 gram
1 pound	=	12 ounces
2.2 pounds	=	1 kilogram

Answers

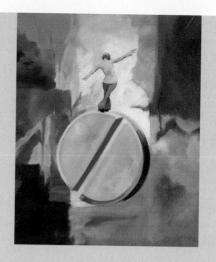

CHAPTER 1
History of Pharmacy Practice

ANSWERS TO CHAPTER REVIEW QUESTIONS

1. d. all of the above
2. a. religion
3. b. materia medica
4. d. 1618
5. b. still used today

CHAPTER 2
Pharmacy Law and Ethics

ANSWERS TO CHAPTER REVIEW QUESTIONS

1. d. autonomy
2. a. FDA
3. b. Durham-Humphrey Amendment
4. b. Class II Devices
5. a. Kefauver-Harris Amendments

6. a. C-I
7. d. adulterated
8. a. 5
9. d. no
10. b. DEA 222

CHAPTER 3
Terminology and Abbreviations

ANSWERS TO CHAPTER REVIEW QUESTIONS

1. b
2. i
3. e
4. a
5. o
6. d
7. l
8. g
9. f
10. m
11. h
12. c
13. j
14. n
15. k

CHAPTER 4
Routes and Dosage Formulations

ANSWERS TO CHAPTER REVIEW QUESTIONS

1. b.   cream
2. d.   lotion
3. a.   bypasses the gastrointestinal system for absorption.
4. c.   lozenge
5. d.   All of the above are true.
6. d.   All of the above should be considered.
7. b.   exits the body quickly after absorption.
8. c.   injected under the skin for absorption.
9. d.   Both a and c are correct.
10. a.   has a longer absorption and distribution time in the body

CHAPTER 5
Anatomy and Physiology

ANSWERS TO CHAPTER REVIEW QUESTIONS

1. b.   homeostasis
2. c.   amino acids
3. a.   outside
4. d.   sugars
5. a.   liver
6. c.   nucleus
7. b.   tissues
8. d.   neurons
9. a.   an organ
10. c.   thrombocytes

CHAPTER 6
Top 200 Drugs

ANSWERS TO CHAPTER REVIEW QUESTIONS

1. c.   heparin
2. a.   USP
3. b.   belladonna
4. b.   USAN
5. d.   all of the above
6. c
7. a
8. e
9. d
10. b

CHAPTER 7
Community Pharmacy Operations

ANSWERS TO CHAPTER REVIEW QUESTIONS

1. b.   nursing home pharmacy
2. c.   the patient walks into the pharmacy.
3. b.   patient's age
4. d.   all of the above
5. c.   verifying the final prescription
6. c.   accept a prescription order by phone
7. b.   check the NDC and/or UPC code
8. c.   phone number of the prescriber
9. d.   the portion of the cost of a prescription a patient pays each time
10. c.   a set fee paid out of pocket before any or full benefits are paid

CHAPTER 8
Community Pharmacy Calculations

PRACTICE PROBLEMS

1. Cost + Markup

   $1.29 \times 1.35 = \$1.74$

2. Price − Cost

   $1.74 - 1.29 = \$.45$

3. $\dfrac{0.4 \text{ ml}}{1 \text{ dose}} :: \dfrac{30 \text{ ml}}{x \text{ doses}}$

   $x = 75$ doses

4. $\dfrac{80 \text{ mg}}{0.8 \text{ ml}} :: \dfrac{x \text{ mg}}{0.4 \text{ ml}}$

   $x = 40$ mg

5. $\dfrac{80 \text{ mg}}{0.8 \text{ ml}} :: \dfrac{x \text{ mg}}{30 \text{ ml}}$

   $x = 3000$ mg $= 3$ grams

6. $0.04 \times 180 \text{ g} = 7.2 \text{ g}$

7. $100 \text{ mg} \times 10 \text{ ml} = 1000 \text{ mg} = 1 \text{ gram}$

8. $200 \text{ ml}/5 = 40 \text{ doses}/4 \text{ doses per day} = 10 \text{ days}$

9. price $-$ cost

    $\$8.95 - \$1.10 = \$7.85$

10. $\dfrac{(\text{Price} - \text{Cost})}{\text{Cost}} \times 100$

    $\dfrac{8.95 - 1.10}{1.10} \times 100$

    714%

ANSWERS TO CHAPTER REVIEW QUESTIONS

1. b.   Young's Rule
2. b.   0
3. a.   1:3
4. b. $18.29
5. d.   69 tablets
6. a.   0.2 ml
7. c.   30.9 kg
8. d.   1390 mg
9. a.   695 mg
10. b.   33.42%

Chapter 9
Introduction to Compounding

ANSWERS TO CHAPTER REVIEW QUESTIONS

1. a.   cost effectiveness, availability, solubility, and stability
2. b.   patient, practitioner, and pharmacist
3. c.   therapeutic care
4. d.   *Pharmacy Times Magazine*
5. a.   pharmaceutical calculations
6. b.   the pharmacist
7. c.   formula
8. d.   both before and after the procedure

9. a.   an emulsion
10. b.   glass

Chapter 10
Institutional Pharmacy Operations

ANSWERS TO CHAPTER REVIEW QUESTIONS

1. b.   monthly
2. a.   OBRA 1987
3. a.   nursing home
4. c.   advisory committee
5. d.   checked by a pharmacist before being dispensed
6. d.   all of the above
7. c.   unit dose
8. d.   all of the above are true.
9. d.   give the OK for medications to leave the pharmacy
10. c.   eye drops

Chapter 11
Institutional Pharmacy Calculations

ANSWERS TO CHAPTER REVIEW QUESTIONS

1. 5 hours
2. 25 hours
3. 4 hours
4. 11 hours
5. 25 hours
6. midnight
7. 6 bags
8. 20 mls/hr
9. 167 mls/hour

CHAPTER 12
Introduction to Sterile Products

ANSWERS TO CHAPTER REVIEW QUESTIONS

1. d. provide personnel with protection from hazardous agents
2. c. preparation of hazardous drugs
3. b. High Efficiency Particulate Air
4. b. 0.22
5. d. intravenous
6. b. colorless
7. b. 7
8. a. strength of the drug
9. c. DNA samples from all employees
10. a. prescription eyeglasses

Index

DUR (drug utilization review), 18, 72
Durham-Humphrey Amendment of 1951, 9
Dusting powders, 58
Dyazide, 112

E

Edema, 41
Education responsibilities in institutional pharmacy, 164
Effervescent tablets, 34, 49–50
Effexor XR, 113
Elavil, 113
Electrocardiogram (EKG), 88
Electrolytes, 34
Elidel, 117
Elimination, 34, 73
Elixir, 34, 54
Emergency medicine specialists, 41
Emergency needs, providing, 163
Emergency-use drugs in prefilled syringes, 191
Emphysema, 41
Emulsions, 34, 51, 55–57
  compounding, 156
Enalapril, 116
Enbrel®, 66
Endocardium, 86
Endocet, 116
Endocytosis, 77
Endorphin, 41
Enema, 34, 53
Energy, conservation of, 76
Enteric coating, 49
Eosinophils, 84
Epidermis, 82
Epiglottis, 98, 108
Epithelial tissue, 78–79, 80
Equipment and supplies
  for aseptic technique, 187–193
    biological safety cabinets, 188–189
    IV bags, 191–193

laminar flow hoods, 187–188
    needles, 189–190
    syringes, 190–191
    vertical flow hoods, 188
  for compounding, 153–154
Errors
  institutional pharmacy as principal defense against medical, 163
  insurance billing, 134
  medication-related, 165
Erythrocytes, 41, 80, 84
Escitalopram, 113
Esomprazole, 112
Esophageal sphincter, 98–99
Esophagitis, 34, 41
Esophagus, 98
Estraderm®, 63
Estradiol, 118
Estrogens, 34, 75
Ethical decisions, 5
Ethics, 5–8
  defining, 5
  moral philosophy and, 5
  pharmacy technician code of, 7–8
  practicing, 6
  theories of, 6–7
Ethics of care theory, 6
Ethinyl estradiol/norethindrone, 116
Euphoria, 41
Evista, 115
Excipients, 154, 158
Excretion, 34, 41
Excretory system. *See* Urinary system
Exhalation, 107
Exocytosis, 77
Expectorants, 34
Expiration date, 130
Extended-release medications, 33, 48, 58–59
External, 41
External aerosols, 58
External powders, 58
External respiration, 106

Extractives, 57–58
Extracts, 57–58
Ezetimibe, 116

F

Facilities, compounding, 154–155
Facts and Comparisons Book, 197
Fahrenheit, converting Centigrade to, 144–145
Faxes, receiving order by, 127–128
FDA. *See* Food and Drug Administration (FDA)
FDCA. *See* Food, Drug, and Cosmetic Act (FDCA)
Feces, 98
Federal Bureau of Investigation (FBI), 16
Federal laws. *See* Law, pharmacy
Felodipine, 118
Fenofibrate, 115
Fentanyl, 117
Fever, 96
Fexofenadine, 112
Fexofenadine/pseudoephedrine, 115
Fibrinogen, 85
Fidelity (moral principle), 5
Filing methods for prescriptions of controlled substances, 18
Filling prescriptions, 130–131, 169–171
Film coating, 49
Filter needles, 189
Filters, 197
Filtration in kidneys, 103–104
Final approval of pharmacist, 131, 169
Finasteride, 118
Fleet® Enemas, 67
Flexeril, 114
Flomax, 114
Flonase®, 63, 113
Floor stock, 167–168
Flovent, 115
Fluconazole, 114

Villi, 99
Vioxx, 112
Virtue-based ethics, 7
Virus, 45
Visceral, 45
Viscous aqueous solutions,
    53–54
Visine®, 68
Vitamin D, 80, 81–82
Vitamin K, 99
Volume, metric prefixes with
    standard measures of,
    205
V-Tids, 114

W

Warfarin, 114
Washes, 53

Water-in-oil emulsions,
    56–57
Water-soluble ointments, 51
WebMD, 204
Weight(s)
    apothecaries', 205
    avoirdupois, 206
    metric prefixes with standard
        measures of, 205
Wellbutrin SR, 113
Wernicke's area, 92
White blood cells, 84–85
    hormones generated by, 96
Withdrawal symptom, 39

X

Xalatan®, 68, 115
Xanax, 112

Y

Yasmin 28, 115
Young's Rule for pediatric doses,
    143

Z

Zantac, 113
Zestril, 112
Zetia, 116
Zithromax, 112
Zocor, 112
Zoloft, 112
Zolpidem, 112
Zyloprim, 116
Zyprexa, 115
Zyrtec, 112
Zyrtec-D, 117